ADVANCE PRAISE

With *Your Energy Signature: A Healing Professional's Guide to Creating a More Powerful Practice* Bear McKay clearly and thoroughly shows us the process of the energetic styles and patterns we each develop. We can have the same patterns, the same character structures, and yet we embody them in a way that is uniquely ours.

I have lived my life supporting others seeking personal and professional growth. As the Founder and Director of The Institute of Healing Arts and Sciences, my world has been filled with energy healers for literally decades. For those of us who chose to bring healing to the world, this work is imperative. How can we heal others if we haven't done our own healing? One thing I have learned over the years as I watched myself and my hundreds of students grow in this work, is that we cannot take others to places we haven't risked going yet ourselves. This work supports you in getting there!

Even after being immersed in this material for over 30 years – and teaching it for 19 - in reading this book I could see things with new eyes. Bear's presentation style, her love of this work and this knowledge, and her ability to combine it all and teach it to anyone is such a joy to experience.

Do yourself a favor. Get this book. Find yourself within these pages. Understand your vulnerabilities, your strengths, your beliefs, and your patterns. The best ending possible is in seeing that ANYTHING can be developed, changed, or strengthened. Bear shows you how

DOROTHY A. MART

PSYCHOTHERAP

"*Your Energy Signature* is an essential handbook for healing practitioners. Bear makes the study of the human subtle body and psychological dispositions accessible, practical and instructive. Her work offers specific insights into the main energy types we each embody and how to bring them into balance so we can benefit from the gifts they each possess. A culminating body of work that no healer should be without."

KATHLEEN JOY, CREATIVE LEADERSHIP CONSULTANT

"A fascinating read and very well written. Healers, practitioners and general readers alike will benefit from this book. The information is valuable on so many levels! To discover your own energy signature is the start of a journey of change and growth; to discover other's signatures is the ultimate in loving and assisting them on their path. I will be referring to this book time and again."

COACH PAULA GROOMS, LMSW

"I highly recommend Bear's informative, clear and very readable book. As a psychotherapist and energy practitioner, I draw from this model of energy patterns in helping my clients discover their gifts and leave limiting habits behind. Bear was one of my early teachers, and I am delighted that she is formally sharing her wisdom in this book. Bear makes energy patterns accessible for the lay person and practitioner alike. This is a fab book which I will be recommending to my clients, supervisees and colleagues. Spend an afternoon reading this book and discover a way to a more vital life!"

KATHLEEN DUNBAR, LMFT AND CERTIFIED
HAKOMI THERAPIST

"Wow! I am impressed. As a massage therapist, I feel *Your Energy Signature* should be required reading for massage students, and if one is already licensed, then as part of license renewal requirements. Knowing energy signatures would help balance the client/therapist relationship, and bring even more benefits to the therapy of massage."

MOLLY BURTON, MASSAGE THERAPIST

"Bear McKay's new book, *Your Energy Signature*, is a pithy, clear and enjoyable ride into finding your type based on energy patterns and body form. You may know yourself through your astrological sign or profile or your Enneagram number, but these energy types are designed to locate you now, in your body, and provide ways to promote healing and growth.

McKay's writing is easeful and informative, and she offers the possibility of health with information that is available to us – right in front of us. Actually it IS us. Our bodies are manifestations of energies that are guiding (running?) our lives. With knowledge and insight into physical and emotional tendencies the 5 types manifest, Bear reveals our old wounds and offers practices, exercises and simple adjustments that could potentially bring us into the balance we seek in this human life.

This slender and helpful book is good for the individual and great for anyone in the helping or healing professions – you can cut through much noise when you ascertain your clients' essential strengths, weaknesses and needs."

KAREN DECOTIS, SOTO ZEN BUDDHIST TEACHER

"*Your Energy Signature* is a great, easy-to-read book that anyone can use. Bear explains what the energy types are and how to work with your weaknesses and recognize your gifts. Learning my energy signature has been life changing for me, personally and in my business. I recommend this book to anyone who wants learn what makes people tick and how to change repetitive patterns that are not working."

RONDA MEYER, MASSAGE THERAPIST

"I loved reading this book – an objective view of our personalities and how we behave and interact with each of the others. It is easy to understand when laid out in this format and allows me to recognize behaviors of others and myself on a deeper level. Especially helpful are the diet and exercise hints for each category, because of corresponding habits we naturally fall into. All people can benefit from this peek into human behavior."

LANI MALMBERG, ENVIRONMENTAL LAND RECLAMATION SPECIALIST

Your Energy Signature

your
energy
signature

*A Healing Professional's Guide to
Creating a More Powerful Practice*

BEAR McKAY

NEW YORK

LONDON • NASHVILLE • MELBOURNE • VANCOUVER

Your Energy Signature

A Healing Professional's Guide to Creating a More Powerful Practice

Published in New York, New York, by Morgan James Publishing in partnership with Difference Press. Morgan James is a trademark of Morgan James, LLC.
www.MorganJamesPublishing.com

The Morgan James Speakers Group can bring authors to your live event. For more information or to book an event visit The Morgan James Speakers Group at
www.TheMorganJamesSpeakersGroup.com.

ISBN 9781683508090 paperback
ISBN 9781683508106 eBook
Library of Congress Control Number: 2017916056

Cover and Interior Design by:
Chris Treccani
www.3dogcreative.net

Interior illustrations by Luz Diaz

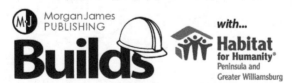

In an effort to support local communities, raise awareness and funds, Morgan James Publishing donates a percentage of all book sales for the life of each book to Habitat for Humanity Peninsula and Greater Williamsburg.

Get involved today! Visit
www.MorganJamesBuilds.com

DEDICATION

To my parents for encouraging me,

my children for motivating me,

and my teachers and students for engaging me

on this path of awareness.

TABLE OF CONTENTS

PART ONE

INTRODUCTION

An Extra-Ordinary Model

This book has been a long time in coming. Yet all timing is divine; over the years, my appreciation for and understanding of energy signatures has only increased through my own life experiences and working with my students. It is now the primary lens through which I view myself and other people. It's how I minimize my inherent liabilities and strengthen my natural abilities and gifts. I have learned from many teachers – and have lots of techniques and models to work with as an energy healer – but this is the one model that puts all the pieces together and gives them coherent meaning. It is a working model that has changed my life and those of my students and clients. The perspective of energy signatures has made me a better healer and teacher, and a way better spouse, mother, daughter, and friend! I accept and view others from a deeper level of understanding. It has softened my judgment;

because of it I am more compassionate toward others. I can give and receive more freely.

You don't have to "see" energy to assess someone's energy signature; the body has all the information you need to start with. The physical body is our densest energy body and it shows you how the energy is patterned. You only need to know what to look for. Broad shoulders, defined facial features, the shape of the torso, the eyes, limbs, and posture all have a story to tell. A few questions can further refine that determination. If you are in a healing profession, notice how your client interacts and responds to you as a practitioner. Are they spacey, acting helpless, charming, intimidating, do they try to reverse roles and take care of you? As you work with them, why does a particular technique help one client and not another? What is the deeper pattern behind their presenting complaint? What approaches can you take to help them come into balance? The answers to these questions are usually related to their energy signature. With this model, you are immediately on your way to serving that client better, and having a more productive interaction.

There are five energy types – Priest, Lover, Gardener, Warrior and Royal. Our energy signature is a combination of two major types plus a third minor one. Each one impacts our thoughts, feelings, behavior, and health more than you could imagine. You will make some adjustments to your evaluation as you work with someone and get to know them better, but the first glance is usually pretty right on. In the individual chapters on the energy types, you will find a physical description and the attributes that indicate the major patterns of each energy type.

This book is my gift to you. Bold and revolutionary thinkers and observers of the embodied human experience have made it possible. My contribution as a teacher is to simplify and make complex ideas and practices accessible. This model works. So start with this understanding and apply it first to yourself, then to your loved ones and clients. Get familiar with the types that make up an energy signature. There are practices here to begin working with the more negative aspects of your energy signature that are holding you back or even creating disruption in your life. You'll find that energy signatures provide a model for understanding yourself and your clients in a larger context.

You will be surprised at how much it explains!

Adventures in Healing

On my way to becoming an energy healer, I studied various healing traditions, spiritual and religious practices, and philosophical belief systems. As a teen, I tried out Transcendental Meditation and experimented with mind-blowing, consciousness-altering substances. I was reading Alan Watts, Carlos Castaneda, and Black Elk. I sat deeply with the question of "What is reality?" At the same time, I was engaged in finding a form of expression for my experiences in journalism, theater, and film. I am fascinated by the ways in which we as individuals interact with and view the world; how we create our lives, shape our experience, and ultimately, affect our health.

I found myself immersed in that richness as an educational/documentary filmmaker. I loved the experience of being on location, and how people allowed me to become intensely involved in their lives for a short time. It was a deep and intimate glimpse into another's world. Through my films, I wanted to touch others as they had touched me.

While filming in Alaska I found two special mentors – an Inuit healer and a documentary filmmaker. Amos Burg was a filmmaker and adventurer, making movies with a hand crank camera (before the advent of sound recording) in places as far away as China. He was also an outdoorsman and river runner – the first one to go down the Colorado River in a rubber raft (rubber donated by Goodyear, and yes, he filmed it!) He was self-educated, dropping out of school and going on an ocean voyage as a young teen; he read the entire Encyclopedia Britannica on that boat. He was in his 80s when we met and spent time together. After a lifetime of adventure in the natural world, he told me, "The next great explorations will be those of the inner worlds."

Whenever I asked about a native healer in Alaska, the answer was always the same – Della Keats, or "Puyuk." I searched her out in the northwestern village of Kotzebue, and we became fast friends. I decided to make a film about her – after all, I was a filmmaker! – and in the meantime, she was showing me all kinds of healing techniques. (She knew what I was supposed to be doing long before I figured it out.) Her story started when, as a young girl, she miscarried at three months. In the midst of winter, camped near the Noatak River, she kept the fetus alive in a cardboard box positioned high in the tent. By turning this tiny being every few hours – he would flatten out – and feeding him drops of animal butter, he survived (he was in his 40's when I met him). She went on to become a renowned healer, using traditional Native means and also through her intuitive sensing. She was open to and eager for any kind of healing knowledge. She explained her gifts as God-given, and yet practiced alongside Western medical doctors when they arrived in the Arctic. She told me how to undo a cord wrapped around a baby's neck while still in utero, move a breech baby, realign a shoulder, and use a certain healing plant as a medicine and in spiritual ceremony. She performed amazing feats of healing, both mundane and miraculous. Her advice to me – over and over – was to "learn everything, from anyone you can!"

I pursued energy healing in earnest when I became stuck in my patterns and life became unbearable – in an unhappy marriage, my work dead-ended, bored, broken, and hopeless. I took out the garbage one day and saw myself taking the garbage out every Thursday and then dying. I was renovating my garden at the time, and when I went to the lumberyard I saw a tree graveyard; at a landscaping supply place, I saw stones that had been ripped from their native homes. I felt pain for the earth when a highway I traveled on had been cut through a hill. If I had seen a mental health professional, I'm sure I would have been diagnosed as clinically depressed. I was lost and searching for a meaning to my life beyond the mundane: a way to express myself in the world that was satisfying and contributed to the greater good. The answer was clear to me once I looked over my bookcase and saw what my true interests were – healing, religion, philosophy, and the nature of consciousness.

Over the next three years, I completely transformed my life – ended my marriage, trained in energy healing, and moved from San Francisco to Montana with my two young daughters.

I was excited about life again, and my adventures with the world of energy and healing were just beginning.

Inspired by Amos I have explored the inner frontiers of energy and matter as it relates to healing and the human experience; and through Della's influence, I have strived to learn everything I can, from many great teachers. Some of these teachers are in physical bodies, some are energy beings or guides, and some of what I teach has arisen in the context of my interaction with a client. I have drawn on Western, Eastern, and indigenous models of healing.

If you are in a body, you have work to do; but it gets easier, life gets better, and the work with your energy signature becomes more subtle. New layers emerge; knowledge becomes embodied wisdom. I don't know how I would have gotten through all those difficulties that comprise a life without it. I am endlessly fascinated and engaged with my process and those of my students and clients. I hope you are, too!

The Ghost in the Machine

D o you ever wonder exactly how the "mind-body-spirit" connection works? What are the specifics – the mechanisms – for the interrelationship of these aspects of our Being? How do we understand and work effectively with this knowledge to improve health and well-being for ourselves and for others? What if you were aware of the unconscious energetic patterns arising from the deepest soul level and manifesting in beliefs, behavior, personality, emotional tenor, defensive hot buttons, interpersonal dynamics, and physical health? Going beyond the concept that *everything is connected* to a practical framework is the basis from which you can heal.

Philosophers from Plato to Aristotle to Descartes (the "father" of Western philosophy) have struggled to understand the relationship between the body and the soul, the physical world and consciousness. Cartesian dualism of the 17th century

11

was popularized by the phrase "the ghost in the machine" – the body being the machine. Stemming from that mindset, no wonder we have a mechanistic view of the body! We see our bodies as a compilation of parts and processes that can be broken and fixed. This kind of thinking has created a fragmented approach to health and healing. We prize the intellect and its discrimination, breaking everything down into the smallest parts possible, including the human body. We see each symptom as something that stands alone, in isolation from the rest of our Being.

More and more evidence is coming forward about the direct connections between body, mind, and spirit – and the impact on our physical health (which is when most of us start to pay attention). While we may theoretically understand that all aspects of our Being are connected, the solutions that Western medicine offers generally address just one symptom or condition. Often the treatment snowballs, treating side effect upon side effect. On a more positive note, supportive therapies are often recommended such as diet, exercise, physical therapy, and psychological treatment – each provided by a different specialist. We run from one appointment to another, trying to take care of ourselves. If an issue is chronic or undiagnosed, we may go from one specialist to another searching for an answer.

Our healthcare system does not support holistic treatment, yet people looking for relief are willing to spend their own money on treatments not covered by insurance (to the tune of $33.9 billion in 2007). As people recognize the limits of the Western medical approach, they are voting with their dollars and their lives by using alternative and complementary therapies. Yet the same fragmentation can happen in alternative and complementary healing; we might seek the help of a shamanic practitioner, an energy healer, a somatic therapist, a chiropractor, a massage therapist, or an N.D.

Think about it; how many health professionals do you consult with? Most people are much more proactive about their health these days, doing their own research and trying different practitioners, supplements, diets, and exercise programs. We try to understand our health issues from myriad perspectives but often get conflicting advice. It is frustrating when no one we consult with addresses the complexity of who we are and what may be the origin of our ill health. We are masters of dissection, but what connects and animates all these disparate parts? It is the connective tissue of spirit and energy that we in the West don't understand very well.

As unsatisfying as our current model of healthcare is for a patient or client, it is equally if not more so for many health practitioners. Those of us who enter into healthcare and healing professions usually do so out of a genuine concern for others and a desire to help. Nonetheless, it is not very satisfying to treat the same presenting complaint over and over again, while the real cause is left untouched. The underlying reason for a condition often creates the same or similar issues again in the future. Physical symptoms are the tip of the iceberg; the ultimate causes are deep underwater and can be as varied as the individual. That's why a particular approach may work well for one person, and not at all for another.

Having one area of specialty with its narrow focus limits the nature of the treatment modality with a client. The interaction between practitioner and client typically revolves around this focus. Many factors that could be influencing the condition are not explored. We as healers yearn to make a bigger impact – to address the source as well as the symptoms of health issues. There are many integrative techniques that can be learned and folded into a practice that help expand the effectiveness of healing work – the bigger the toolbox the better. Yet tools are in service of a larger perspective. Spontaneous intuition may help guide your healing work, but results might still be spotty without having a comprehensive model and context to work from.

Having a practice where people are looking to you for help is very satisfying when you are successful. Yet often the success is short-lived. The frustration of not being able to make a bigger difference, coupled with the boredom of a narrow focus, can make it difficult to stay the course. Eventually a practitioner might become disengaged, feeling ineffective and uninspired, or even overwhelmed by a client's needs.

As a practitioner, you could be noticing energetic interactions between you and your clients that are puzzling. Most of the time people are not conscious of energy dynamics, but know that there is something going on. Body workers can literally pick up energy from their clients; some even feel physical sensations such as pain or constriction in the same area the client is experiencing it. Long term, these are not viable ways to practice. Following a routine, numb to the possibilities, can lead to burn out. Understanding and working with energy signatures can help practitioners avoid these unhappy scenarios.

It Starts With You

What if you had a road map of your client that directed your focus and helped you connect the dots between the myriad aspects of their experience? What are the different dynamics that contribute to the client's set of issues? What if this same map influenced how you approached and worked with them to get the most effective outcomes? What if every session, even with the same client, was different and interesting? What if you got amazing results with your practice and had a fuller, richer relationship with clients? What if you could continue to work with people no matter the diagnosis or other ongoing treatments?

It's possible to be refreshed and satisfied with your work. If you are curious about the unique nature of the person you are treating and how the pieces of the puzzle fit together, you can continue to be challenged and deeply engaged with your work.

While you might still refer out to other health professionals or work in conjunction with other healthcare modalities, you can continue holding the space for your client to be seen in their entirety. You can help integrate the results from other healing work and mitigate side effects of traditional allopathic treatments.

Clients will keep coming back and be willing to pay you more for your attention and comprehensive approach. I do a lengthy intake asking about many things – not only physical history (from birth on) but family and relationship history, lifestyle (diet/digestion, exercise, sleep, feminine cycles, medication, and supplements), spiritual practices, other approaches they've tried, the current concerns, and what was happening in their lives at the time of the original incident or onset. People are incredibly moved that a health professional is taking the time to ask such a deep variety of questions and to truly listen to them. Viewing people and ultimately yourself from a more holistic perspective tends to create more compassion for the human condition – challenging, joyful, and mysterious!

It's easy to learn techniques for pushing and pulling energy, releasing blockages, and increasing energy flow without any self-awareness; often I see healers that seem to be completely clueless about their own energy patterns. Learning how to perform an energy technique is a skill and a starting point. How much energy is being sent, what is going on boundary-wise, where the energy is going, and how the client's physiology is responding are also critical to know. As healers we are not just *doing* something to someone else – it is an interactive collaboration. The healer supports the best possible health for the client, which is different for every individual. You can't just make things happen through your will and skill. Being attached to an outcome will create issues for you and is not your job as a healer.

A healer's awareness and level of consciousness plays a big part in their capacity to heal – and the client is affected by resonance with the healer's energy field. When you truly understand the nature of healing, you recognize your potential impact in the role of healer. It is an honor, privilege, and responsibility to work with people in this intimate way. You have gratitude for the amazing results of the work, and are humbled in the face of a greater intelligence – and the connectedness of all things.

Start with yourself; after all, we are the subjects we are most fascinated with! Your life is a learning laboratory, offering up many ways to pay attention and develop a new way to approach an issue. Any good healing school will involve quite a lot of self-healing and self-analysis. That's the good news; we are always a work in progress. Once you start down the path of healing, the growth never stops. Fortunately, you don't need to reach a level of perfection to be a great healer. We are all wounded, with the inborn capacity to heal ourselves and others. Healing is not a solitary endeavor, though; no matter how adept or conscious we are, we all need support, community, and love in our lives.

Knowing your own energy signature can be a tremendous help in how you work with clients; understanding your client's energy signature can determine how effective your treatment is. Although energy healers have many ways to bring more balance to energy signature patterning, this model can be applied by any health professional – in fact by anyone – to improve their lives, their health, their relationships, and their work.

4

Standing on the Shoulders

I teach many different models and techniques for healing, from Eastern, Western and indigenous origins. This particular model comes from Western psychoanalytic theory and was created by Wilhelm Reich. He called it "character analysis" and, in more recent times, it is known as characterology. Reich was a visionary who initially was a protégé of Freud; he was a rising star in the psychoanalytic world of Vienna in the 1920s. It was during this time that he developed his model of character types. He elaborated on these major psychological patterns that arise from developmental crises, create a self-fulfilling belief system, drive defenses and emotional armoring, and shape personality. He named the types after the developmental wounding – Schizoid, Oral, Masochist, Psychopath, and Rigid. (Sound like fun?)

As he became more radical in his thinking and theories, he fell out of favor in community after community, moving from Germany to Norway and finally to the United States. The truth is he was bat-shit crazy, and a genius. He died in prison at the age of 60 after the FDA brought him to trial for his "orgone energy" generators. Ostracized by his peers, he was a man ahead of his time – but one with serious personal issues. He talked about orgone and orgasmic energy and (like his mentor, Freud) was fascinated with issues of sexuality and genitalia.

Two of Reich's students continued to develop ways of working with the characterological types. Dr. John Pierrakos and Dr. Alexander Lowen devised one of the earlier forms of mind-body psychotherapy called Bioenergetic Analysis. John and his wife Eva, who wrote many volumes of channeled guidance, founded a spiritual community called The Pathwork Center. John also developed another offshoot of character analysis and created The Institute of Core Energetics in 1973. Reich's work also influenced many of the New Age therapies of the 1970s, including Gestalt therapy and Primal (Scream) Therapy.

Others have continued to develop the model, most notably Barbara Brennan. She wrote *Hands of Light*, the seminal work on energy healing. After several years of private practice, she started the Barbara Brennan School of Healing in 1982. She was introduced to Reich's model through John Pierrakos, Core Energetics, and the Pathwork community. She noticed the chakra dynamics that correlated with each energy type, and wrote about characteristics of each type in a less psychoanalytic way. Her significant contribution to the model, along with an energy healing perspective, was to widely introduce the characterological model to a new audience.

Another innovator, Ron Kurtz, expanded the model as well. He founded a "body-centered psychotherapy" program called Hakomi. He co-authored *The Body Reveals – What Your Body Says About You* with Dr. Hector Prestera, which details the types and even defines sub-types. Many others, including Anodea Judith and Dorothy Martin-Neville, have written about this model within a broader healing context.

My personal linage of teachers for this model includes Barbara Brennan, and later her student Michael Mamas. (I graduated from his School for Enlightenment and Healing in 1998.) I studied briefly with John Pierrakos and Rosalyn Bruyere, a teacher of Brennan's. In my early days of practice, I became familiar with the Hakomi training when I had many of those practitioners as energy healing clients and students. I discovered that many people who have been introduced to the model were not fully utilizing it. Therefore I have drilled it into my students – because it is a comprehensive overview of who we are in the world, how we came to be that way, and how we can change for the better.

I introduce the energy signature model right away in my program and teach to it in every single class throughout my curriculum. It is layered, complex, and nuanced, and it is helpful to have support as you work with it personally and professionally. Teaching it in layers is less overwhelming and more digestible. Time and practical application make it an invaluable resource.

One simple change I made had a profound effect on my students' ability to work with their characterological types – I renamed the types to reflect their gifts. At first I kept the old psychological names in parentheses. I didn't want people to think they could just manifest the gift without working through the wounding – no one gets off easy here! Even so, the original names got in the way. It could take a long time for someone to fess up to being a masochist or psychopath – and several months to a year before they could start working with the model productively. The minute I renamed them, they could embrace their energy signature right away. We have a lot of fun with our types, laughing at our foibles and frustrations. If you don't laugh, you will cry, because you will come to understand more deeply your suffering and the suffering you have created (unconsciously) for others. We can't escape the human condition of suffering, but we can come to terms with our past transgressions and forgive ourselves, forgive others, and be a better person – and healer – moving forward.

PART TWO

Energy Patterns and Energy Ruts

Life is a combination of free will and destiny. We are born fresh, and a baby *seems* like a blank slate. A look at how unique each baby is in body, temperament, and needs tells a very different story. Although babies can't communicate through language, they carry many lifetimes of stories and patterns. We arrive in this world with a predisposition to a particular energy signature in order to fulfill our destiny. Each life event and circumstance begins to shape and create a particular path – a life story. As we get older our responses and decisions seem to define our lives more and more narrowly. Yet in the beginning, our defenses and strategies for getting what we need served us. Later on, the dark side of these patterns comes into play. When we are unconscious, unaware, and reacting, we keep re-creating our worst fears and scenarios. We can feel this stuck-ness; an energy pattern becomes an energy rut, predictable and demoralizing. For many this becomes a (quarter-life? mid-life?) crisis – change or die! Yet even within the same circumstances of our lives, there is the possibility of spaciousness, of liberation from the prison of our ingrained way of being.

How do we change and grow? The first step is learning and awareness, and we have the intellectual learning part nailed. The second step is integration of this knowledge, which is essential but the part we are not so fond of. For instance you could read this book, and then thinking you have learned about your energy signature, put it down and keep on doing "that thing you do!" Nothing would change. Sometimes we take multiple classes or trainings and yet nothing seems to make a difference. You may learn new techniques for your healing practice and, after the novelty wears off, never use them again – or, when an appropriate occasion arises, you wonder, "How did that go again?"

Intellectual learning is Doing. Integration demands Being, enabling us to live what we have learned. In our culture we are intensely focused on doing, growth, increase, more, more, more. We judge others and ourselves by how productive we are; we value busy-ness. This addiction has created a huge imbalance in how we live in the world. We have a serious Being deficit; the mindfulness movement is speaking to that need, and we are thirsting for meaning, peace, and contentment in our lives. Less *is* more, but we rarely act that way.

When we are in the Doing state we are active; Being is the state where we receive, we listen, and we sense energetic information. Appropriate Doing arises from Being. The key to healing is being able to move back and forth from Doing to Being freely. In child development, the theory that there are periods of growth followed by periods of integration – the experiential aspect of learning – has gained acceptance. How often do you know what to do – in terms of diet, exercise, a supplement regimen, meditation – and are not able to actually do it? We tend to judge ourselves when we aren't able to do something right away and give up, maybe rationalizing that our failure is due to the inadequacies of the program or class or teacher. The real issue is the difference between superficial study and actually being able to implement that knowledge in your daily life.

The old way in education was to stay with a subject until it was pounded into your head through memorization. Learning done like that can get you through a test but often doesn't stay with you. In the spiral model of learning, you touch on subjects for awhile, not waiting to completely "get it," then move onto another concept, re-visiting the initial subject material later. The learning happens in stages – it has time to sink in and be connected to the whole, and when it is studied again it is from a deeper level. Lasting growth happens only when you take time to integrate what you have learned. Along with our Being deficit, we lack patience with the integration phase. It can feel like a plateau where nothing is happening, but it is critical to real change. Integration – learning through practice – is the way we transform rote knowledge into embodied wisdom.

Everything is just practice! I love the word practice; it takes the pressure off. You are simply *practicing* new behaviors. You might recognize you have launched into a habitual pattern, like a knee-jerk defense or poor boundary, after the fact. After several hundred times, you will eventually notice *before* it is about to happen – and still won't be able to stop yourself! Congratulations, you are in the next phase of your development. After several hundred times of this "premonition," it's possible to occasionally experience a space – or gap – between pattern and action; it is in this gap that we can choose another way. Not every time, but with practice, we are no longer compulsively driven by our extreme patterning. As you engage in this process, practice becomes ever more subtle, and eventually the old constraints are just ghost patterns that barely register on your consciousness. Awareness, learning new skills, attention, and practice all lead to the integration of a new pattern. This need for integration is just as true for the physical body as it is for behavior and beliefs. When as an energy healer I introduce a change in the physiology, the tendency is to revert back to the old patterning; new ways of being have to be continually re-introduced for them to finally "stick." Don't be discouraged; your patterns will become less extreme and more modulated over time. You will move into the territory of responding rather than reacting. We are big on learning and changing and growing but don't give ourselves the space for integration. Be patient with yourself and your clients, allowing your efforts to germinate and flower into a new life.

All change requires effort: the initial effort to learn something new, and then, most importantly, the awareness and effort to put it into practice. As we notice and practice, something important is happening underneath: growth in consciousness.

Energy Signatures in Action

Since our energy signature is made up of two major types and a minor third, the interplay between our types can be quite variable. You may find a situation where an energy type shows up that is not in your signature at all. (Surprise!) It could be that with one person, or in one kind of interaction, you exhibit the patterns of an energy type not in your top three – or even your top four. Likewise, if you are confused and think you are ALL the types, just take it one situation at a time. Investigate your responses, your behavior, and feelings in that particular context and work with the presenting energy type no matter how it plays in your signature. It will be much simpler to work with one of the types in your energy signature at a time.

There are stages of life that are influenced by certain energy patterns but don't determine an individual's signature. Children exhibit Lover qualities (so sweet, so clingy); Gardener,

Warrior, and Royal patterns are noticeable in mid-life when we are working to build families and careers; and old age is characterized by a withdrawal into the more spiritual nature of our existence (Priest).

The energy types will combine in different ways for every person; for instance a Warrior-Gardener may have a very open 5th/throat chakra (Warrior) or very little energy moving through the throat area (Gardener). Once the energy signature is assessed, the variations unique to that person can be determined over time. After all, models try to approximate and explain reality, but we are much more than a model and models *are not* reality!

You may notice one of your types seems dominant in a given context. Often there is a work life/personal life split in how the energy types in your signature come into play. One of your major types may operate in the personal arena and the other in the work setting. This is why people can be confused, for instance, about their boundaries – so clear and strong at work, and non-existent in intimate relationships. It is easily explained after understanding the types that make up a signature. So notice when one of your types arises more strongly in a particular context and just work with the dynamics that are in play at that moment. Don't think that flipping between your energy types is any kind of workable compromise! One student was a push-over boundary-wise (Gardener) and when she had enough, she would aggressively take charge (Warrior), leaving her co-workers totally confused. Two extremes of patterning do not create balance.

People wonder if there is a "perfect" type to be, thinking that they may be able to change their type. You develop the major energy types of your signature at an early age and these will always be your energy types – your areas of focus in personal work, and your innate talents. What *can* change is becoming more balanced in your patterns so that your gifts manifest in a bigger way. What holds us back are the original beliefs we developed and the resulting energy patterns that are excessive or extreme. The goal is not to change our signature, but to realize our gifts more fully.

Sometimes people think the Royal is one of the best types to be because they are so amazingly productive! Like all the energy types, there is a downside involved and once you fully understand the Royal's suffering, you will not think being a Royal is ideal. Likewise there is no perfect kind of spouse, employee, co-worker, or friend; it depends not so much on their type but on how balanced they are in their patterning. Even so, knowing energy types and signatures can lead you to hire people with an eye to their strengths, making everyone happier in the roles where they can shine.

You may have noticed that siblings are usually very different from one another. Just because you have parents with their particular energy signatures, it doesn't follow that all the children are certain energy types. We come into this life pre-disposed to a signature based on what "assignment" we have chosen for this lifetime. A baby may be left alone in its crib while mom takes a shower for ten minutes; one infant can be completely engaged, infatuated with its toes, while another experiences abandonment. These responses speak to their inherent energy types, which direct their development and the strategies they use to adapt to family circumstances.

There is no perfect energy type for a spouse! It doesn't follow that "x" type will be best off with a "y." Remember, it's a combination of energy types that makes up our signature, which would complicate such a simple formula. I have noticed when two people have the same energy type within their signature it can help, as there is an unstated understanding between them (and then again, opposites do attract!). Differences in tidiness, organization, finances, and child-rearing that come up in a relationship can be traced to each person's energy signature. Understanding your partner's energy signature is very helpful in creating a harmonious household.

Again, if it sounds too complicated or confusing just start working with one of your types that shows up in a particular context or with a certain person and go from there. You will grow in your understanding and awareness as you notice and practice!

7

Your Energy Signature – The Quiz

First, put a checkmark next to descriptions that are true for you; choose as many as you want. Count up the checkmarks in each category (A, B, C, D, and E.) Rank the categories from the most checks to the least.

The top two checked categories are your major types; the next one is your minor type.

If you are older, base your answers on yourself at mid-life; if you are younger, remember that many health conditions don't develop until later in life.

A.

My physical characteristics are:
_____ thin
_____ one shoulder/hip higher
_____ one leg/foot turns out slightly
_____ loose-jointed
_____ spinal curvature

My health concerns are:
_____ spinal curvature
_____ joint problems
_____ nervous tension

When stressed I feel:
_____ scattered
_____ overwhelmed

When asked to do something I:
_____ need to check and get back to you

My personality is:
_____ spiritual
_____ creative

TOTAL CHECKS: _____

B.

My physical characteristics are:

_____ thin, slightly longer arms

_____ sloping shoulders

_____ forward pelvis and/or head

_____ big eyes

_____ full lips

My health concerns are:

_____ autoimmune issues

_____ fatigue

_____ hormonal balance

When stressed I feel:

_____ emotional

_____ collapsed

When asked to do something I:

_____ only want to do it if others are there too

My personality is:

_____ sweet

_____ nurturing

TOTAL CHECKS: _____

C.

My physical characteristics are:
_____ square torso
_____ dense musculature
_____ compact neck
_____ shorter waist
_____ tucked pelvis

My health concerns are:
_____ digestion and assimilation
_____ problems in the throat area
_____ reproductive issues

When stressed I feel:
_____ buried
_____ shut down

When asked to do something I:
_____ commit no matter how inconvenient

My personality is:
_____ easy going
_____ constant

TOTAL CHECKS: ____

D.

My physical characteristics are:

_____ broad shoulders

_____ chin up

_____ chest forward

_____ smaller calves

_____ large hips/thighs (for some women)

My health concerns are:

_____ kidney issues

_____ high blood pressure

_____ shoulder problems

When stressed I feel:

_____ angry

_____ critical

When asked to do something I:

_____ do it if it serves/interests me

My personality is:

_____ charismatic

_____ forceful

TOTAL CHECKS: _____

E.

My physical characteristics are:
_____ symmetrical shape
_____ tense muscles
_____ rigid neck
_____ straight, tight back
_____ well-defined facial features

My health concerns are:
_____ heart disease
_____ stomach issues (e.g. acid reflux, ulcers)
_____ headaches

When stressed I feel:
_____ anxious
_____ dissatisfied

When asked to do something I:
_____ will do it if I am available

My personality is:
_____ active
_____ detail-oriented

TOTAL CHECKS: _____

The top two checked categories are your major energy types; the next one is your minor type. The combined types are your energy signature. If you are confused, read over the descriptions of the types and see what fits you best.

A) _____ Priest

B) _____ Lover

C) _____ Gardener

D) _____ Warrior

E) _____ Royal

My top 2 (major) types are:

_____

_____

My next (minor) type is:

_____

8

Defining Elements of the Energy Types

The following overview will help orient you to the descriptions of the energy types. Although I have separated out these elements, they are all ultimately interrelated. Working with one element or area will actually help you in some of the other areas – we build health synergistically, not in a linear way. For instance, you can't completely resolve all your boundary issues without addressing beliefs, and you can't change your physical health without working on the chakras. They all work together, but you can't work on them all at once. Pick and choose what is most important for you to get started.

Physical Health and the Body

The body is energy made visible. Areas of greater or lesser energy flow show up as differences in size, shape, and density. Health is greatly affected by the main energy imbalance; where the energy flow is too high or too low in an area, or there is compaction, troubles are bound to arise. Early development and beliefs also help shape the body's form (i.e. "there is not enough" produces a concavity in the chest area indicating lack; the "I need to be perfect" produces external symmetry and tension; the "not wanting to be seen" results in literal obscuration/padding of the torso.)

Energy Metabolism

Energy metabolism describes the way and rate at which energy moves through the body. It has to do with density and the chakra baseline, and our metabolism impacts the overall energy available to us on a daily basis. It influences the way we digest food and process emotions. Our energy metabolism is also affected by those around us, especially when weak boundaries are in play. Diet, exercise, how we structure our activities (even sleep), and who we choose to surround ourselves with are all ways to mitigate our too slow or too fast energy metabolism.

Energy Flow and the Chakras

The main energy imbalance can easily be assessed – whether left/right, top/bottom or internal/external – when you know what to look for. Energetic defensive patterns help create and reinforce these imbalances, which will become more exaggerated over time if not addressed.

The chakras are seven areas centered down the midline dynamic of the body that draw in energy from the environment, including other people. Along with food, it is the energetic nourishment that sustains us. Each chakra is associated with a physical system and psychological and emotional issues as well. The activity of a chakra also affects the nearby organs and the area of the body it is located in. For instance, an overactive 3rd chakra (solar plexus area) affects the stomach even though the system it relates to is muscular. Low energy in the 2nd chakra (abdominal area) will affect digestion, but is also directly related to the reproductive system.

Everyone has a chakra baseline – some chakras having less flow and some more, and some may be *too* open or active. In addition to this baseline, the chakras' degree of openness will reflect the situation or context. Some chakras will naturally be more open in a business meeting; other chakras, when you are being intimate. The idea that all chakras should be wide open simultaneously is a fallacy, and is quite uncomfortable should they be forced open. A good healer will work on balancing the system as a whole, gently and over time. Big changes arbitrarily forced on the chakra system or other energetic structures cannot be integrated. While this may feel cathartic and dramatically different for a client, the artificially induced changes do not last. The system will on its own contract back down to the normal baseline.

About Chakra Energetics

In the Appendix is an exercise called Chakra Energetics. This easy ten-minute exercise encourages a subtle opening of your chakra system and is of benefit whether you practice it occasionally or on a daily basis. It's fun to do (kids of all ages love to join in!) and helps you feel grounded and invigorated. I have seen it help with depression, which is a lack of overall energy in the system.

As you go through a series of sounds and movements for each chakra, you are actually generating the frequency of that chakra. You can do the whole exercise quickly, but it's interesting the first few times to stop after every chakra and sense into the "field" or frequency that you have created. Notice which ones you like, which ones feel like home, and which ones might be less comfortable. The description of the exercise also includes specific characteristics of each chakra: the color/frequency, governing attributes and issues, and the physical system it is related to. This is a good way to get familiar with the chakras and I have all my students memorize this simple chart. There is a lot of information available on the chakras – it's an energy map of the physiology that is thousands of years old! – but you can keep it simple for use in everyday life.

In the sections that address how to balance your energy type, I have listed which chakras are compromised for that type. Do not focus just on those chakras with this exercise; it could cause too rapid of an opening, making for some discomfort. It's best to work with the system as a whole.

Early Development and Beliefs

We all develop strategies for survival as infants – ways to get what we need from our parents and our environment. The most basic human need is love, and to be safe and protected (and fed!) through that loving relationship. The family we are born into is never perfect, and based on what we experience (along with our predisposition to an energy signature), we develop beliefs and expectations about the world. These beliefs are mostly formed from birth to age five and set the stage for the rest of our lives. "Mirror Mantras" are statements that challenge these unconscious beliefs that drive so much of our experience. Speak these out loud in front of a mirror and repeat until you are convincing!

Defenses and Boundaries

When we feel threatened or our needs are not being met, defensive patterns activate to counter the situation. These defenses are very specific in nature. The pattern becomes habitual, and to a great extent, determines our boundaries. We have the boundary of the physical body, and our energetic boundary is the edge of our auric field. Generally the auric field emanates three feet out from the body in an eggshell shape. This energetic real estate is ours, and, depending on the situation, may be unconsciously expanded or contracted. With a little practice and awareness, we can control our field's size and the amount of interaction we desire. In the auric field we are surrounded by our own personal energetic weather, and other people pick up on variations in our mood and energy partially from our auric field.

Boundaries associated with each energy type are, before any personal work is done, either too weak or too intense. Our energy signature is typically made up of one type from each category, but the combination results in alternating between too weak/too intense boundaries rather than any kind of balance. Equilibrium is the goal, having a flexible but strong and resilient boundary that adjusts appropriately, and allows us to both give and receive. There is also a shape to our boundary that is related to our main energetic imbalance; these distortions will even out as you work with your defensive patterns.

Gifts

Let your soul shine! We are luminous Beings, but layers and layers of patterning obscure the glorious truth of who we are. We inhabit these bodies, created especially for us, to meet the challenges and opportunities of this lifetime. Our strongest gifts always remain those associated with our two major energy types. So by working with the extreme aspects of your energy signature, you free up your gifts and express your strengths in the world. We can transcend our initial limitations and become the Bodhisattvas we were meant to be!

PART THREE

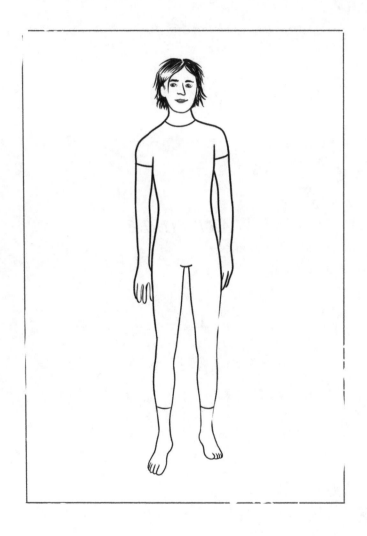

The Priest

CREATIVE, INTELLECTUAL, SPIRITUAL

The Priest is idealistic, quick-witted, and spiritually attuned. They are creative and live very much in the moment. Interested in intellectual pursuits, they question why things are the way they are and how they can be different. They are inspiring and bring new insights into whatever field they are in. They will often choose idealism over pragmatism, as reality is seen as limiting their unfettered dreams and imagination. Their interests are so many it can be hard to focus in any one area, yet when they do, the results are transformative.

Their relationship with time is flexible. They like to be free-form and go where and when the spirit moves them. Time is expanded in the now and there is always enough time, until there isn't! This casual relationship with time leads to always being late and an inability to stay on task or adhere to rigid timetables. They are often in a rush. The ultimate procrastinators, they usually get through a deadline with a burst of energy and focus that is awesome – but temporary. This is problematic in their professional as well as personal lives, and others may see them as undependable. A lack of follow-thru can lead to unfinished projects and unfulfilled aspirations, which discourages these gentle souls and the high-minded ideals they want to put into action.

They crave stimulants (even more than most) because this mimics and reinforces their natural boom-bust cycle of energy. Their minds are razor sharp and focused on the upside – but they are exhausted and spaced out after coming down from the high. One incredibly productive day can be followed by a day spent staring at the walls. They have a hard time maintaining consistency with their activity; any routine schedule, even eating at regular times, can be a challenge. They will forget to eat until they realize they are starving.

Priests have flexible joints and are limber but don't have much endurance for aerobic activity; in fact they are not that physically oriented, mostly living in the world of the mind and ideas. Their dress is casual, unstructured, and creative. They either have a lot of fun with their appearance or don't pay any attention to it at all. An overall left-right imbalance can be noticed by one shoulder and hip being slightly higher than the other; in extreme cases there is significant curvature of the spine. If they are physically active, their left/right imbalance will create a host of joint problems. Typically they will need to force themselves to do the minimum exercise necessary to stay fit and generally don't derive pleasure from physical activity for its own sake.

With the preference for less structure and more freedom, the Priest often falls into the "spiritual not religious" category but takes their spiritual life quite seriously. If they do belong to an organized religion, they tend to relate to the more direct, mystical aspect of their religious heritage. They are apt to be meditators who enjoy Being more than Doing. When out in nature, they would much rather lay in a meadow watching the clouds than climb to the top of the mountain.

Easily bored with details, and loving of distractions, they can have trouble coming down to earth and dealing with the mundane. This lack of embodiment means they often start a project with enthusiasm but don't have the stamina to make it a reality. Money matters don't interest them particularly; like time, there is always enough until there isn't. When circumstances are difficult, they become overwhelmed and fearful, withdrawing when it all becomes too much. They retreat from the harshness of the physical world into the comfort of the energetic and spiritual realms.

Witty, creative, a bright light – the Priest is a lively and deep thinker, pondering the bigger issues, and with a decidedly spiritual bent. Their deep spiritual nature lends itself to religious, philosophical, and artistic professions or outlets. Quite intuitive and innovative, they will surely be thinking along the cutting-edge in whatever field they choose. They are very open-minded and can entertain all possibilities, so much so that it can be hard to choose a course of action. They will generally have lots of projects going on at the same time.

They frequently look off at the horizon while in conversation, as if they were drawing their thoughts down from the ether. Sometimes they can seem spacey, flaky, or scattered. Their desk is a usually mess, but it's organized chaos – they know where everything is! They create out of the intuitive flow, where everything is constantly in metamorphosis.

Priests are dreamers and often unrealistic and naïve. They can find themselves unwittingly involved in dubious situations because of poor judgment or discernment of others. They always want to believe the best about people. Delightful to be around and wonderful companions, they are enthusiastic and charming party guests!

IF ENERGY TYPES WERE ANIMALS…

The Priest is a Giraffe

A Priest has their head in the clouds, most at home in the intellectual, airy realms of ideas and creative impulse. Quick to startle, and fleeing from the slightest indication of danger, the Giraffe's long legs make for a fast escape. Viewing the world from great heights, with a transcendental perspective, the Priest/Giraffe is sustained by the refined atmosphere of the energetic and spiritual realms.

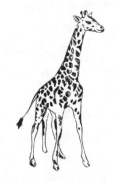

DEFINING ELEMENTS OF THE PRIEST

Physical Health and the Body

The Priest body is generally thin and flexible. Their flexibility is not true muscular flexibility; it comes from being loose-jointed, which makes them quite limber but also susceptible to joint issues. A lack of symmetry between the left and right sides is why an exercise regimen such as running will wreak havoc on their joints. They look like they should be well-coordinated but are actually a bit clumsy, to the point where they can "trip on air." They don't get much pleasure in physical activity just for the sake of it. They are attracted to individual exercise regimens that have a strong internal component, like yoga or swimming, or that are more free-form, like dance movement. Touch, whether personal or in the context of deep massage and bodywork, creates comfort and connection for them in the physical body.

Energy Metabolism

The Priest has a high energy metabolism; the energy whooshes through them and that is why they don't have a lot of physical stamina. It's the reason they can eat like a horse and not gain weight! The brain uses the lion's share of our food energy and the high level of nervous system activity consumes all those calories. They tend to go for quick energy sources like sugar and caffeine, which mimic their boom/bust energy cycle. Many small meals high in protein help to modulate the energy flow in the Priest. This fast metabolism and boom/bust cycle can be seen in their ability to focus: they go from a hyper-alert, focused, and brilliant state, where they are highly productive, to an almost stupor-like lethargy or brain fog.

Energy Flow and The Chakras

The main energetic imbalance in the Priest body is left/right; this is often seen in some form of spinal curvature. It can be detected by a higher shoulder and hip on one side. There is usually a more subtle forward/back aspect to the twist as well. This creates more stress on the hip joints; the forward one gets "crunched" with all the weight thrown on it, and the one higher and toward the back acts as the lynch pin of support for the whole body, and is stressed by keeping opposing forces of motion stable. The left/right imbalance translates from the pelvis and hips into the rest of the leg – knees, ankles, feet. You will often see a Priest putting most of their weight on one side, standing asymmetrically.

The lower chakras, associated with the physical body, are weaker. The 1st (base) chakra is connected to the skeletal system, another reason why bone health can be such an issue. Bones are the densest part of the body and create our physical structure.

The 1st chakra is where we access our primal energy for survival in the physical world. The Priest doesn't want to be constrained by the physical body, being much happier in the worlds of creativity, ideas, the intellect, energy, and spirit. Maintaining a strong heart connection with those they are close to is important. It helps bring them into their bodies and experience being safely held by others in a loving relationship (this includes animals!).

The upper chakras, more associated with energy and spirit, are well developed, and may even be too open and overused. The 6th (brow) chakra, sometimes called the third eye because of its relationship with intuition, rules the nervous system. Priests tend to run on nervous system energy versus physical energy, and they go through regular cycles of intense activity and burn-out. The stress on the nervous system can make them susceptible to, and exacerbate, many health issues.

Early Development and Beliefs

The Priest often enters the physical world with some difficulty in gestation or at the time of birth. This earliest experience leads to a deep unconscious fear of being in a physical body in this precarious world. The world is viewed as a dangerous and even hostile place. The safe world of the womb, or even earlier in the world of spirit, is most comfortable for them. Not being well integrated in the physical body will of course lead to more accidents, which reinforces the belief that the world is not safe! Priest children are dreamy and may have a lot of imaginary playmates, and they are often happy playing "alone" when in fact they are engaged with a fully realized alternative reality.

Priests can be so present with an activity that it is hard to shift gears, yet they seamlessly shift from one idea to the next and are easily distracted. It makes it difficult to conform to the expectations of the rational world of schedules and linear thinking. These are the prototypical ADHD kids – really smart but totally "unmanageable!" Ironically they can be oblivious to their surroundings, and yet keenly aware from an intuitive and energetic standpoint.

Defenses and Boundaries

At the first sign of conflict, the Priest retreats to the world of spirit and energy. If possible they will physically retreat – they just leave. Even if they stay physically, they have exited energetically to the realms where they feel safe. This mild dissociation makes a scary situation tolerable for them. It's the primary defense in the unpredictable world that they find themselves in; even without direct conflict the Priest can feel overwhelmed by the demands of life. This ease of movement between the physical and energetic worlds makes for very weak or even non-existent boundaries! Like the ocean tides flowing back and forth on the shore, it's hard to define an exact boundary with so much movement between land and sea. This affects all kinds of boundaries – time is elastic, money flows in and out, and in conversation and relationship, they are all over the place. Present one moment and then gone the next, they can be easily taken advantage of when they aren't really present. They love the feeling of an expansive energy field, and extremely *permeable* boundaries are a result of their flowing nature.

Gifts

Priests are so fun to be around: creative, full of new ideas, and unconcerned with conventional ways of being. They definitely "think outside the box" most of the time. Their quick wit and intelligence are brought to bear on every subject, and they are excited about the endless possibilities inherent in any situation.

Their biggest challenge is to bring these ideas down to earth: to pay enough attention to one thing long enough to see it through to completion. Manifesting in the physical realm is grunt work for a Priest – they would rather someone else follow through on the details. The deep spiritual connection they experience is a great solace to them. Sometimes referred to as "old souls," they are compassionate, understanding, and tolerant. They are versatile and adaptable; in fact they thrive on variety.

IDEAL ABODES OF THE ENERGY TYPES...

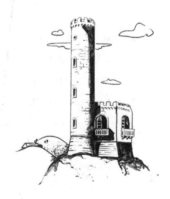

The Priest would retreat to a lofty Ivory Tower for contemplation and creation. Away from the everyday world and maddening crowds to a place of eternal beauty and timelessness, the Priest reflects and designs in complete freedom. Observing the weather and the comings and goings of the people below, planning for the future with intuition and foresight, the Priest spins prophecy.

BALANCING THE PRIEST

Healthy Guidelines

- Weight training for bone strength
- Pleasurable free-flow aerobic movement
- Massage and bodywork, especially Rolfing
- Time-outs with hot baths and resting in nature
- Minimize stimulants
- Frequent high protein meals
- Eating lunch before 1pm
- Bone and nervous system supplements
- Routines for eating, exercise, and sleeping

Chakra Focus

- Chakra Energetics: especially the 1st (base) and the 4th (heart) chakras
- Relax the 6th (brow) chakra– allow intuitive information to *come to you* rather than *seeking it out*
- Bring energy down from the 7th (crown) chakra, through the midline dynamic of the body, between the legs and into the earth

Mirror Mantras

- "I am safe"
- "I am here"

Boundary Work

Visualize contracting your auric field eggshell down to a few feet from your body; this creates more density in the field and the boundary naturally becomes stronger and more defined (pretend you are in "elevator mode").

Literally keeping your feet on the ground while sitting helps!

When lying down, straightening your head if it angles to one side (DO NOT angle it in the opposite direction to counterbalance.)

Antidotes to Defensive Patterns

Don't physically leave when difficultly arises (unless both parties agree on a time out!).

Maintain eye contact (you don't have to gaze or stare) while interacting with people; notice the tendency to look up and away while speaking.

Building on Gifts

The Priest's main challenge is MANIFESTATON. Being in the body and working through the mundane details of the physical world is key to bringing all those great ideas into reality. The best types of jobs involve creative thinking and activity, and allow for periods of freedom to explore these energetic realms. This free time combined with incremental deadlines (preferably imposed from outside) helps the Priest be at their best; being held in a routine by others is a recipe for success. A balance of collaboration and solitary time helps stoke and fuel the generative fires.

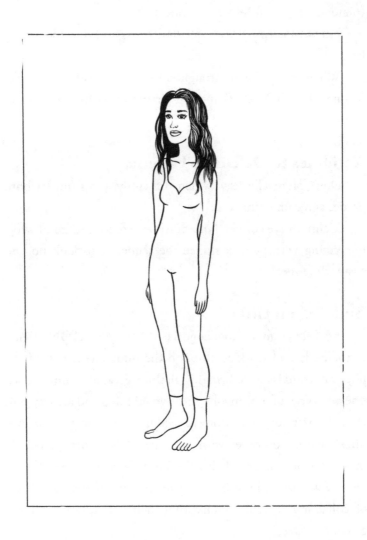

The Lover

SWEET, NURTURING, SENSITIVE

The Lover is the ultimate nurturer – sweet and caring, they naturally gravitate toward others and are attentive and altruistic. Instinctively knowing others' needs, they make great parents and teachers. They always want company but can be happily engaged in independent activity if someone else is nearby; they appreciate the presence of others. This makes them very social – whether introverted or extroverted they like to be in a crowd. In conversation, they might find it hard to disengage. They give a lot but expect to be attended to in return. They don't have much physical stamina, but depending on their other major type can happily participate in group athletic activities if they are so inclined. In their spare time, they like to be pampered and to pamper others. They

61

easily blend in or take on the opinions of a group in order to be to be a part of the action.

The blessing and the curse of the Lover is their extreme sensitivity. Both internally and externally, they notice subtle movements of energy and are aware of the slightest disturbances in "the field." If they read about an ailment, they immediately sense in to see if they have it, and often can find evidence for it. This makes them the hypochondriacs of the energy types! Understanding their sensitivity and accounting for it can help them be realistic about their health.

Their sensitivity can lead to feeling hurt by stray comments or opinions that are expressed with less than tact or diplomacy. They extend this sensitivity to others' feelings as well and are able to point out an injustice to others or explain another's injured response to a situation. They can act as a social conscience in a group, and would be great in leading sensitivity trainings for business. They are very considerate and caring and would never hurt a living being; they are the ultimate peacekeepers. Placing this importance on the welfare of others (as well as themselves) they can imagine, and help create, a world of peace and harmony. They are gentle souls.

Lovers can feel abandoned at the slightest infraction or disagreement. When facing a loss, the Lover can become needy and clingy. Ironically, this pushes people away and manifests their own worst nightmare – being alone. When threatened, they will either take what they need or simply give up, feeling hopeless. Often they give up before they even try. In their worst moments, they can become hysterical when they feel abandoned or discounted.

Physically they seem fragile, and this fragility is emphasized with big eyes and soft voices which make others want to care for them. They can easily feel hurt and may need consistent reassurance to keep moving forward with a project, but are generally delightful and a people pleaser – very unthreatening. Sensual in nature, they love to eat, drink, and even smoke. They eat for pleasure, and that includes eating with others. Typically thin, sometimes they have a protruding belly when they are older.

They dress well and are usually quite attractive and even flashy, which brings them the attention they crave; they spend a lot of time on their appearance. The attention they look for is more personal than professional, based on who they are rather than what they Do. Like a beautiful flower that attracts the honeybees, they simply *are* in the world.

For a Lover, spiritual teachers are preferable to a rigid ideology; they may be drawn to bask in the glow of a guru. They are great helpmates as long as they are paid enough attention. They can become exhausted by too much responsibility but will willingly follow a lead, as long as they are not left alone to do the job.

IF ENERGY TYPES WERE ANIMALS...

The Lover is a Monkey

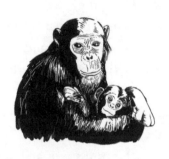

The Lover is captivating, inviting, and offers loving attention. With big eyes and lips, they are very expressive and want to interact. They can spend hours grooming one another and are very concerned for the emotional welfare of the group. The Monkey has long limbs that make them very adaptable, at home on the ground or in the trees. The Lover/Monkey is a social animal, perceptive and endearing.

DEFINING ELEMENTS OF THE LOVER

Physical Health and the Body

The Lover tends to be thin, and often their arms are a bit longer in relationship to the rest of their body. The first thing you notice about them is their beautiful engaging eyes. The slightly rounded and/or sloping shoulders are protecting the heart area, and there may be a noticeable concavity in the chest area. A soft voice tends to draw people in and it can be difficult to extricate yourself from them in conversation. Overall they have less strength and physical stamina than other energy types. A lack of energy creates a susceptibility to autoimmune diseases. Constant internal checking and their ultra-sensitive natures lead them to always noticing what could be wrong or is missing. Their sensitivity – external and internal – is both a blessing and a curse.

Energy Metabolism

The overall low energy level of the Lover means their metabolism will be sluggish. It takes them a long time to get going. They feel more energized in groups and love social gatherings. Uneven energy levels will have them questioning their health, and looking at diet and other external or environmental factors to explain their lack of energy. For the Lover there is never enough of anything, including time, energy, and money. Ironically, they will often leave food on their plate because an empty plate is the worst case scenario – there is nothing left! They will want back-ups of back-ups in the food pantry, just in case…

Energy Flow and the Chakras

The main energetic imbalance is internal/external, with less energy internally. They are then looking outside themselves for what they need and don't feel very full or satisfied on their own. This is why they prefer company to being alone. The chakra system and midline dynamic are undercharged overall, especially in the 4th (heart) and 5th (throat) chakras. These two areas are concerned with receiving nourishment of all kinds – food, love, and energy.

Early Development and Beliefs

There was some lack of nourishment in the early months of life; perhaps it was literal, if they were on a strict feeding schedule, but it could also be attention – babies thrive on attention and touch as well as food. When breastfeeding, there is more going on than mother's milk; her gaze and the interaction are just as important. The lack may not be obvious, as a parent can be distracted or not fully present when they are with the baby. There could be other small children in the house that need consideration, or a difficult situation in the family. Whatever the reason, the Lover feels short-changed and has two main responses to this: they either give up without trying (because they won't get what they need anyhow) or they actively try to get attention and energy from others. They can alternate between these two strategies.

Defenses and Boundaries

In giving up, the Lover collapses and this closed energy field can be a precursor to depression. When distraught, this collapse becomes hysterical, which ironically is the fastest way to clear a room! Their other defense, to look to others for energy, can manifest as clingy behavior. Both of these defenses cause people to withdraw, reinforcing feelings of abandonment and making things worse. The boundaries of a Lover are very *enmeshed* with others, as there is a lot of both give and take in their interactions. This is a weaker boundary that gets more defined when they have a stronger sense of self in relationship.

Gifts

It is interesting that, while they didn't receive the love or nourishment that they needed when young, Lovers are the most naturally nurturing of the energy types. The sweetness they exude is hard to describe. While the Gardner and Warrior will Do for you, the Lover will Be there for you. They are very empathic and truly feel for others, without taking on the emotions and energies of others. They are excellent spouses and parents. (Male Lovers are often the parent a child will go to for comfort.) They are best when working in a collaborative environment, surrounded with people who have the same concerns and values. They add a personal touch to everything they do that makes them stand out. When balanced, they feel full on their own and aren't excessively needy. Lovers bring an incredible sensitivity to any situation; they are often the ones to alert others as to how they might be affecting someone else adversely. They are a great asset for keeping a team in alignment and identifying when values are being compromised.

IDEAL ABODES OF THE ENERGY TYPES...

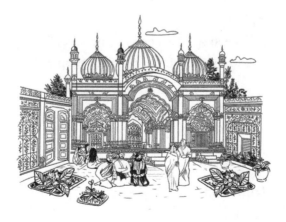

The Lover would inhabit an Indian palace with its intricate, delicate, and sumptuous architecture and decoration. Life in the palace, with a large extended family, is a constant unfolding of sensual and culinary delights within a web of enduring relationships. Beautiful gardens and a large kitchen producing the most delicious, tantalizing food complement the fullness of life in the palace.

BALANCING THE LOVER

Healthy Guidelines

- An emphasis on good posture; build upper body strength
- Exercise with a buddy
- Completely finish food and drink
- Discover and utilize your homeopathic constitutional remedy
- Endocrine system supplements, especially adrenal supplements
- Meditate in spiritual environments and groups
- Have a solid healthcare team for support

Chakra Focus

- Full chakra energetics exercise: especially the 4th (heart) and 5th (throat) chakras

Mirror Mantras

- "I am full"
- "There will always be enough"

Boundary Work

Visualize a little sun in your solar plexus emanating out and filling your body, then filling your auric field.

Don't immediately ask for help; notice this tendency and check in and see if it is something you can do for yourself.

Antidotes to Defensive Patterns

When feeling weak or going into an emotional collapse, visualize a line of grounding energy from the 3rd (solar plexus) chakra down between the legs and into the earth.

Bookmark any situation in which you feel full or satisfied, with as much sensory detail as possible; recall this feeling when experiencing a sense of loss or "not enough."

Building on Gifts

The Lover's main challenge is INDIVIDUATION. Lovers shine when they feel sufficient, even powerful, unto themselves; it's the key to consistently receiving the attention they desire and being sought out for their sensibilities. They are excellent teachers (especially of infants and young children) and caregivers, and have a calm and reassuring presence. They work best with others or on a team, and have a keen understanding of emotional dynamics; they will be the first one to notice if someone is hurt and will attend to that person. Their sweetness and attention to others makes them the best – well – lovers!

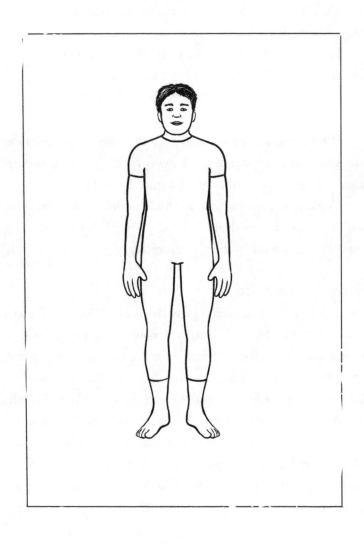

The Gardener

EMPATHETIC, STRONG, GENEROUS

Gardeners are the engines of the energy types. They have a lot of physical endurance and are most comfortable serving others, preferably behind the scenes. Their efforts make everything happen; they are the gears and cogs of human machinery. They are wonderful spouses, family members, and friends, putting their self-interest aside to help others. Generous to a fault, they will go out of their way to be helpful – even to the detriment of their own health.

Others' needs take priority, but if they are not appreciated or acknowledged in return, they will become resentful. They don't often express these feelings but pack away the grievances until they have an explosion, usually reserved for those closest to them. Then it's back to the happy-go-lucky, super-helpful, always-there-for-you, lovable person. They anticipate what others need, often volunteering before being asked. Be aware that they have unspoken expectations for their efforts, even if it's as simple as considering them a good person.

Subordinating their own needs and feelings becomes a real self-care issue eventually. Although they are incredibly strong and grounded, eventually (in mid to late life) they will burn out. Packing in their needs and feelings – which they may barely be aware of – becomes literal weight. They carry around emotional baggage, theirs and other people's, in the form of pounds. They are the drama queens (and kings) of the energy types, but it is usually OPD (other people's dramas). They will insinuate themselves into situations where they can be the heroic helper.

They have problems asking for or expressing what they want, but will expect you to know anyway – by either reading their minds or by picking up on an extremely subtle hint. Not wanting to draw attention to themselves, they will rarely speak out. This can be exasperating for those close to them – they don't express how they feel or what they think. If they have a physical complaint, they won't "bother anyone" by communicating about it, and often they aren't aware of a physical issue until it becomes unmanageable. This leads to serious health problems not being addressed until the last minute.

They are capable of intense physical labor but don't necessarily engage in sports because of getting plenty of activity at work. Slow and steady will always win in the end in terms of getting the job done. They are great workers and don't need credit – as they like to avoid the spotlight – but do like to be appreciated.

They go over in their minds what they should have, could have, would like to have said in a given interaction and can keep a grudge alive for a long time. They may act like a doormat but don't take them for granted! They are passive-aggressive and you will pay for your transgressions (often with no idea of what you should have done, since you didn't read their minds!). Along with being the masters of passive-aggressive behavior, they are stubborn as all get out. They will rarely say no but will sit and stall – it's not happening, but they will never tell you so.

Although they can be large and seem intimidating, they are big teddy bears and are responsive to others' energies. Being so tuned into others, they can actually take on other people's feelings and even physical sensations. Their self-identity lies in helping others, and this lack of self-esteem leads to enabling others but ultimately resenting it.

IF ENERGY TYPES WERE ANIMALS...

The Gardener is a Bear

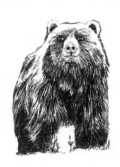

The Gardener appears soft and cuddly but be forewarned – they are a strong and powerful force that you don't want to cross! There is beauty in their economy of movement, and their endurance is legendary. They are good providers and have deep inner resources that get them through periods of difficulty like a Bear in hibernation. As they are a fearless protector of those they love and a fearsome enemy, pay attention to the subtle signals of the Gardener/Bear.

DEFINING ELEMENTS OF THE GARDENER

Physical Health and the Body

Gardeners have a square torso (no matter how much they weigh) and are compactly built. Their physical density gives them enormous reserves of strength and endurance. That is a good thing, as they continually push themselves to Do more! Their hearts are actually larger than average, which speaks to their generosity. The density of their bodies can create sluggishness in digestion and overall metabolism. It takes longer to process food, emotions, and toxins, while exercise only slightly improves their ability to assimilate. Given the fact that they tend to take on others' energy and emotions as well, it can be a lot to process. Holding on to energy and dispersing it slowly creates a build-up within the system. The neck is often short or thick which also leads to congestion in that area. Heart disease, digestive problems, and throat conditions – including thyroid problems – are what they need to look out for.

Energy Metabolism

The slow energetic metabolism is responsible for weight gain over time. Gardeners can exercise and eat one salad all day and still gain weight! Addressing the hidden reason for weight gain is essential to health because the weight puts even more pressure on a hard-working heart. Yet the Gardener doesn't like to let things go, whether it is excrement, sinus or throat mucus, toxic emotions, or a silent grudge. (They need to learn to let go of feelings in little amounts of titrated expression. Depending on their age, they may have a huge backlog.) Emotions are released when you enter into them fully, which allows them to move and transform – the Gardener can do neither.

Energy Flow and the Chakras

The main energetic imbalance is internal/external. The Gardener tends to hold onto things longer than necessary, packing them away to be dealt with – or not – at a later time. The internal environment is quite compacted, and the energy flow is from outside to inside; but somewhat like a black hole, some things never escape! A Gardener *can* move things through their system, but it takes a lot of effort, considering all they have taken in and on. In order to hold in their own emotions the energy is congested at the 2nd (abdominal) and 5th (throat) chakras, effectively closing down the openings of the torso "container." Occasionally the 1st (base) chakra is also affected. There is also less energy flow at the top of the legs, in the groin area. Their internal awareness is not well developed because of this density, so health conditions can get out-of control before they notice anything is wrong. This lack of attention to themselves and bodily sensations means they typically have a high tolerance to pain. This, coupled with the lack of self-care, can lead to a health crisis.

The lack of flow in the 5th (throat) chakra inhibits not only expression but the ability to give and receive deep nourishment – whether it is food, or love (remember those lips are more than the starting point for the digestive process!). They even have difficulty accepting compliments. Gardeners need to remember that Doing is only one part of a relationship.

Early Development and Beliefs

In the "terrible twos" stage when a child starts to assert a sense of self in the quest for independence, Gardeners were met with a controlling and invasive authority figure (often a parent). The message that meeting the parent's needs was more important than their needs leads to a lifetime of taking care of others without considering themselves. Perhaps they had a sick parent to care for or were an older sibling who took care of the younger children. In all these cases, the message was that they are not important. The feelings that arise – anger, resentment, hurt – are not acceptable to have, much less express or acknowledge. This is a real violation of selfhood. They have difficulty receiving praise or compliments and yet are unhappy when they don't get acknowledged for their contributions. It is ironic that they are the ones who create this situation by not wanting to draw attention to themselves! Hoping that others will intuit what they want, they don't verbalize their needs; if they actually say something it is the slightest of hints that many people don't get. (They expect other people are "reading" them as they do others.)

Defenses and Boundaries

The main defense of the Gardener is to take it on, hold it in, and ignore it. They have *accommodating* boundaries which change depending on the needs of others. A boundary this flexible and elastic is bound to be weak in nature. They will appear submissive in order to be accepted and loved. People can smell this a mile away – they will zero in on them at a gathering and proceed to tell them all their troubles. The Gardener is in danger of being a dumping ground for other people's "stuff." With such poor boundaries, they can actually feel other people's emotions and physical pain. No person can take on this much! To regain equilibrium, the Gardener will have an explosion of emotion, a real doozy of a meltdown. They are like a pressure cooker, building up steam and then releasing it in a big burst. Once they explode, they go back to the old pattern of taking on and packing in, and the cycle begins anew.

Gifts

Gardeners literally have a huge heart for a reason – they are the most giving and generous of the energy types, providing essential support for others. When they take care of themselves and are liberated from needing constant approval, their true nature of caring compassion can shine through without any unspoken strings attached. Their care for others is more often expressed in a one-to-one relationship rather than toward a bigger group. They are a marvel of staying power and are the best friends and workers, and are masters at materializing in the physical world.

IDEAL ABODES OF THE ENERGY TYPES...

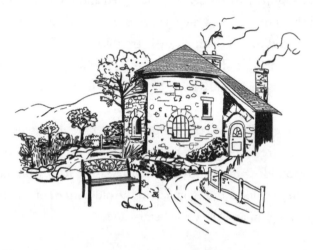

The Gardener would be cozy in a Hobbit house, a cottage that is close to the earth's grounded energy and fertility. Responding to the seasons, the cottage can be shuttered and the hearth stoked, or the windows wide open with sunshine and climbing trellises adorning its entry. The cottage is always well stocked, for the Gardener works hard to produce an abundant harvest; guests are always welcome to share in the bounty.

BALANCING THE GARDENER

Healthy Guidelines
- Create a regular routine of self-care and prioritize it; attend to your needs *first*
- Exercise with a focus on stretching

- Aerobic exercise (being physically active at a job does not count)
- Experiment and find a way of eating that works for you *all the time* instead of bouncing on and off diets
- Digestive supplements such as probiotics, enzymes and triphala (an ayurvedic herbal formula)
- Make sure you have at least one bowel movement a day
- Liver and endocrine system supplement support
- Singing!!!

Chakra Focus

- Chakra Energetics: especially the 2nd (abdominal) and the 5th (throat) chakras
- Sensing into your 4th (heart) chakra, visualize a line of energy moving up and out the front of your 5th (throat) chakra, especially before difficult emotional communication (practice this first in less stressful situations)

Mirror Mantras

- "I am important"
- "I want to be seen and heard"

Boundary Work

Practice the word *no*. Say no to requests for help and then notice – do you relent right away? Feel guilty? Minimize your needs in the situation? Being aware of this self-talk will help you eventually develop good boundaries. Also, notice when you volunteer without being asked; are you trying to curry good favor? Ingratiate yourself? Want something (unspoken) in return?

Disengage from the "takers" in your life. You can still love them, from a distance…

Antidotes to Defensive Patterns

Cry a little, laugh a lot, express yourself along the way before you build up anger and resentment. (Watching dramatic movies is a way to get started…)

Clearly communicate your requests and priorities – no hinting or thinking "they should know!" Notice the small things that irritate you and investigate what's under that anger.

Journal to start to develop internal awareness. Bodily sensations, emotions, and thoughts – which are often the forerunners of emotion – are all game. (As well as other people! You don't have to be nice in your private journal.)

Building on Gifts

The Gardener's main challenge is FREEDOM. The Gardener feels burdened by their duty to put others' needs first. They then try to get their needs met surreptitiously – unspoken contracts like "If I do x for you… then you will do y for me" come as quite a surprise to the other party! The Gardener has a lot to give and are the big hearts of the energy types, but only when they come from a place of having their own needs met can they give generously without any strings attached. They are enthusiastic team players and are best acknowledged for their efforts in a one-to-one, personal way. They have deep reservoirs of physical stamina and cheerfulness that make them indispensable to any enterprise.

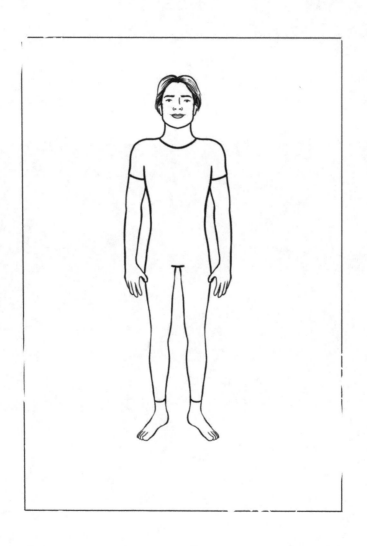

12

The Warrior

INDEPENDENT, COURAGEOUS, RESPONSIBLE

The Warrior is the leader of the pack and is uncomfortable in any other position! They are generally charismatic and are willing to take on risks and responsibility. Ambitious, big picture people, insightful visionaries and entrepreneurs, they are willing to go where no man (or woman) has gone before. They believe in themselves and are confident even in situations where others might question themselves and their abilities. Their way is the right way – and their position is generally summed up as "my way or the highway!" For a Warrior, being right is a question of survival. They demand loyalty and return it in spades; just don't question them or their methods, because they will punish those who betray them.

They are the best boss when they invite collaboration yet are also decisive; give people credit and feedback before re-assigning them; can accept that there is more than one way to achieve any goal; and affirm and bring out the best in their team. They make the worst boss when they aren't self-aware – controlling, micro-managing, and never able to take criticism, no matter how constructive. They can bully and be aggressive; their feedback can be experienced as harsh. As far as they are concerned, they are telling it like it is – and can't understand why people can't just take it. Another way to look at it is that they are blunt and to the point. They have no difficulty expressing themselves and communicating in a direct fashion. If they are angry, you know it immediately, but afterwards they let it go. They may become wary but don't hold onto a grudge unless it's perceived as a personal insult. They will always take up the challenge of a duel, and even enjoy sparring, but you'd better be ready for a few injuries! When two Warriors are in a group they will instinctively fight for dominance.

What would the world do without Warriors? They trust in their abilities and assume it will all work out in the end. Naturally more egocentric than the other types – to lead you have to have confidence in yourself – the Warrior may not be caring in a touchy-feely way but are more altruistic. They care very much about humanity and their tribe, but are not as concerned about individual welfare or feelings. They even minimize their own feelings, and are reluctant to share them. They will express themselves and their emotions intensely if they feel safe enough to be vulnerable, but don't hold your breath. They like to be in control.

People literally look up to them, no matter how tall; they have big energy, especially around their upper bodies, an almost magnetic attraction centered on their eyes and around the head. They may seem larger than they actually are – they appear "bigger than life." Their dress can be dramatic and flamboyant, as they have no difficulty expressing themselves. Charming and seductive, they are very persuasive and enjoy having influence and power, but they do need to keep their ego in check. They don't believe other people will do anything as well as they can, so when they think they are giving constructive feedback or instruction it is often perceived as critical or judgmental. They see their job as taking care of others but are very independent and don't like or ask to be taken care of. Their biggest challenge is to have faith – in others, and in a higher power.

With lots of stamina they tend to push themselves in all settings, including physical activity. They thrive on competition – surprise! – and can power through any activity or demand by sheer force of nature and personality. They enjoy attention and admiration but don't need it – just following their lead is enough. (They like to be challenged by situations and responsibilities, not by individuals.) In their faith groups they will take on responsibility either as the main teacher, leading smaller groups, or being in charge of an area such as finances or special projects. If more generally spiritual, they like to learn from others, and based on that knowledge, originate new practices that they can call their own.

IF ENERGY TYPES WERE ANIMALS...

The Warrior is a Lion

A Warrior has big energy, and the first thing you notice is their mane and their roar! Ready to pounce at a moment's notice or languish about in the dust for long periods, they do as they please as Lord of the Jungle. The Lion saves their

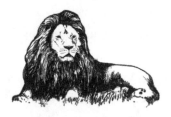

resources for a short intense sprint and then shares the spoils of their conquest. When the Warrior/Lion senses danger from afar, they guide and protect their pride.

DEFINING ELEMENTS OF THE WARRIOR

Physical Health and the Body

The upper body is larger; even Warrior women tend to have broad shoulders (with the exception of the Warrior/Gardener woman, who has large hips and thighs). The contraction on the backside affects the kidneys and low back; the heart is under a lot of pressure due to all the responsibility the Warrior takes on. Developing the lower body through exercise helps support the rest of the physical structure. The shoulders are prone to become frozen because of overwork and taking on too much responsibility. They shine in competitive sports and enjoy the teamwork that goes along with it (as long as they are the captain!). They are not driven to exercise obsessively, nor do they avoid it; it is a part of the bigger arena in which they play. The lack of bulk in the lower legs can lead to knee, calf and ankle injuries.

Energy Metabolism

Warriors can push through anything; while they can keep up this performance, it will eventually take a toll on them. They carry a big load but make an effort to take care of themselves, too. They need substantial food but, more importantly, the time to relax and savor it; they are one of the energy types that find it especially hard to receive. They enjoy large dinner parties and being social with their guests and are more often than not the hosts.

They are gamblers and risk takers with their money, time, and energy; willing to bet on themselves – even though they are not entirely sure they can pull it off – they usually do so through sheer willpower (and bluffing!). They extend themselves, endlessly, but when things don't work out, they go into hiding as failure is unacceptable.

Energy Flow and the Chakras

The main energetic imbalance is top/bottom. The upper body carries more energy than the lower half, and is actually physically larger through the shoulders. The lower half of the body is noticeably smaller, especially from the knees down. It is surprising to see skinny toothpick calves supporting such a big upper structure! Another minor imbalance is between the front and the back. The chest is thrust forward, which creates a stronger arch in the low back and contracts the backside of the body. The chin and head naturally tilt up, increasing the contraction in the back of the neck, too. The contraction on the backside especially affects the rear aspect of the 4th (heart) chakra and these muscles are quite tight.

Their gifts as teachers and leaders are evidenced by a very open 5th (throat) chakra. This speaks to their skill in communication, and assimilation and integration of information into a coherent strategy or plan. The 1st (base) and 2nd (abdominal) chakras tend to be lower in energy, just as their physical body is smaller on the bottom half.

Early Development and Beliefs

As a young child, around age three or four, the Warrior was asked to, or decided to, step into responsibilities more appropriate to an adult. This can be for many reasons: a parent, usually of the opposite sex, is absent from the home through divorce or travel; perhaps a parent is sick or disabled, or simply not present and engaged. The Warrior child can be asked to step into the role of "mommy's little man" or "daddy's little girl," in a subtle way taking the place of the missing or disengaged parent. Taking on these responsibilities at such an early age makes the child feel overly responsible, and the need to be right becomes critical. What will happen if they cannot follow through? Needing to be in charge to assure the well being of everyone can lead to excessively controlling behavior. The world will fall apart if they can't take care of things; their way is the right way, whether it is the best way or not. Being right becomes a survival issue. Their willingness to step in, lead, and take responsibility is courageous and scary – the world depends on them. Failure is not an option. It is a lot to carry. Just as the parent couldn't be fully trusted to follow through, they find it hard to fully trust others. They are unconsciously angry at having to take on so much, but it comes out in many small ways as displeasure and once conveyed is easily dispersed. It's tough being responsible for making the sun rise and set every single day!!!

Defenses and Boundaries

When threatened, the Warrior is like many animal species – they put on a big display of energy, mostly emanating from their upper body. It's how they maintain control and get others to comply if being charming, seductive, and capable doesn't work. Their defense of throwing energy around can be quite intimidating, especially if they are angry and aim those bolts of energy directly at you! Their auric field is larger at the top than the bottom, and their energetic boundary is *aggressive.*

Trying to control every situation is their main defense against the lack of trust in others. They don't believe they have support (they didn't when they were young) and have a very difficult time asking for help, more than the average person. It's as if needing or wanting help is a sign of weakness. They are fiercely independent and want to appear in charge, needing nothing and no one. They are the control freaks of the energy types.

Gifts

Their willingness and ability to take charge and be responsible is a real gift to others; every group needs a leader, and a balanced Warrior considers their role as one of many, all of whom are essential to success. The Warrior needs to learn to relax and trust others to do a good enough job, and to curtail the impulse to take away a job from someone and do it themselves. They are magnanimous, see the big picture, and are visionaries and thinkers, leading the way in many fields of endeavor. They are more likely to be entrepreneurs, given their independent streak and their need to be in charge – they don't suffer fools and don't like taking orders. When allowed to lead, or at least be independent, they really shine. They like to be appreciated and have no small ego (you need one to be in their position) but tempered with humbleness, humility, and an appreciation of the competence and skill of others, they can lead everyone to greatness.

IDEAL ABODES OF THE ENERGY TYPES...

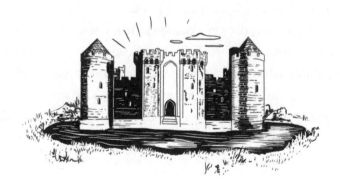

The Warrior would lead from a castle, gathering resources and planning for the future, striking into action when necessary. Always on guard for the enemy and well-fortified from assault, the Warrior takes others behind the castle walls in times of trouble and ensures their safety. Strong, capable and confident, concerned for the welfare of others, the Warrior is not afraid of risk and guides the way.

BALANCING THE WARRIOR

Healthy Guidelines
- A diet that focuses on heart health (including healthy fats)
- Exercise that creates more lower body strength and bulk
- Aerobic activity that is pleasurable and not too stressful
- Massage and bodywork, especially for the shoulders and low back
- Stress supplements
- Adequate hydration and other kidney support; prostate health in men
- Undirected playtime!

Chakra Focus
- Chakra Energetics: especially the 1st (base) and the 2nd (abdominal) chakras
- Communicate with loved ones after sensing into the 2nd (abdominal) chakra

Mirror Mantras
- "I can trust others to do the right thing"
- "I am taken care of"

Boundary Work

Practice letting others be right even though you may have done it differently. Allow others' contributions to be good enough. Find opportunities to say "I'm wrong about that/you're right" and give others credit.

When criticized, don't rationalize; listen deeply and thank the person, then sense into the emotional vulnerability you feel in a private moment.

Antidotes to Defensive Patterns

Visualize dropping energy down from the upper body to the lower body, along with a deep breath, when feeling stressed or angry.

Find ways to physically channel anger – sports are ok as long as you don't get personal!

Stop talking so much…

Building on Gifts

The Warrior's main issue is TRUST and allowing others to do their part without feeling their command is threatened. No one can lead like a Warrior and people naturally gravitate to their circle of influence. Work that allows them to lead and work independently will produce amazing results – trying to constrain them or get them to follow rote rules or policy will stymie their contributions. (Rules are for other people.) They are accountable and always have the big picture in mind, as well as what it takes to get there. They have great vision and understand how to get where they want to go; they can push through any obstacles to be successful.

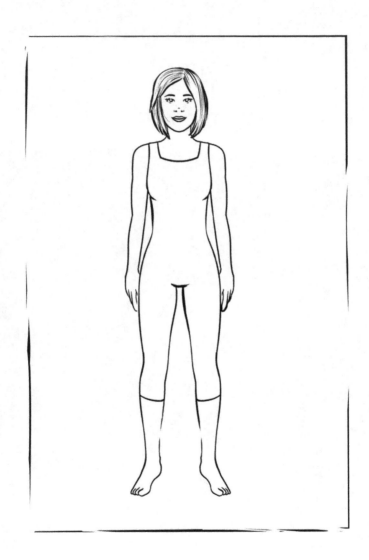

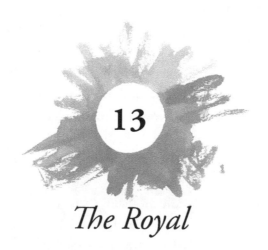

13

The Royal

PRECISE, RELIABLE, ELEGANT

The Royal is a responsible person who likes to get things done. They like clear expectations so that they can perform perfectly; they have high standards and are tireless achievers. Sometimes their perfectionism stands in the way, but they excel at getting things done correctly and are willing to put in a lot of extra effort to get their projects closer to the ideal. They like their work to be recognized and appreciated, but more as positive feedback than from an egotistical standpoint. They want to know they are on track and meeting – or exceeding – the standards set forth. Happy to work as a team member, they will step into a leadership role if necessary (when there is no Warrior in sight!).

They are active and athletic, and like to spend their spare time in physical activity. Their very symmetrical body means they can do many sports well with few injuries. They are as driven in their personal lives as in their professional lives. They go about things in a methodical, organized way – just take a look at their closet! Their dress is appropriate and classic, and they are usually meticulous about personal appearance and hygiene; likewise their homes are orderly and well maintained.

Personally, this excess activity and relentless drive for perfection can take a toll on them, their spouses (unless they married a Royal!) and their families. The emphasis on Doing detracts from quality relationship time and leaves them slightly distanced from their emotional life. After all, emotions can be quite messy and interfere with the schedule! This emotional coolness can be taken the wrong way and seen as hard-hearted. They are never shy about telling people what needs to be done and don't compromise on standards.

They often belong to an organized religion, liking more specific direction and structure even in their spiritual life. They don't mind conforming as they are looking to others to confirm that they are following directives. Given their work ethic, they are often in positions of responsibility, and making money is no problem for them. In fact wealth affirms that they are on the right track. They are organized and plan ahead in their financial lives. They like to be with other Royals who share their standards and have mutual appreciation for all that they Do.

Royals are the ones you want to be engineering bridges, flying airplanes, and coordinating the little league. Other types are envious of the Royal and may be fooled into thinking that this is the best type to be; yet they pay an emotional price for their emphasis on productivity, both in their work and personal lives. The Royal can work 40 hours to get a project 85% perfect, 60 hours to get it 93% perfect, and will continue to put in more hours to eke out a tiny bit more toward the perfect ideal. These diminishing returns for time spent are exhausting and impact the Royal's quality of life. They are rarely satisfied with their performance.

IF ENERGY TYPES WERE ANIMALS...

The Royal is a Dragonfly

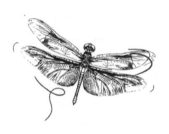

Exquisitely beautiful and delicate, the Dragonfly is also swift, agile and strong enough to travel across oceans. They have a strong exterior of hard plates and they hold their translucent wings out horizontally even at rest. Iridescent coloration and a slim body makes them a standout in the insect world. The flight pattern and movements of the Royal/Dragonfly are complex and precisely choreographed. Their long life span is active and singular.

DEFINING ELEMENTS OF THE ROYAL

Body and Physical Health

The Royal is the most fortunate of the energy types in terms of physical symmetry; they are built for action. And it's a good thing because of their drive to discharge excess energy through physical activity, both task-related and in athletics. Their symmetry allows them to participate in sports with fewer injuries as their bodies are in balance; professional athletes usually have Royal as a main component of their energy signature (swimmers are Royal-Warriors, runners and basketball players Royal-Priests, soccer players, Royal-Gardeners). Their health problems are a product of this over-abundance of energy and driven nature. What we would call an "A" type, they are prone to headaches and stress-related disorders like anxiety. They are also the type most likely to suddenly (surprisingly) drop dead of a heart attack in mid-life. They are wound up and hard-wired. Their muscles, especially back and neck muscles, are very tight. The diaphragm is not very flexible.

Energy Flow and the Chakras

The main energetic imbalance is internal/external; that is, less energy internally in the midline dynamic and more energy on the surface of the body. This uncomfortable surface energy creates tension and a need to release it through physical movement. They also have less energy flow in the 2nd (abdominal) and the 4th (heart) chakra. An overactive 3rd (solar plexus) chakra literally disrupts the connection between the 2nd and the 4th chakras, making it easy for the Royal to compartmentalize love and sex. The excess energy in the 3rd chakra creates stiffness in the diaphragm and often translates into stomach issues such as acid reflux and hiatal hernias. Royals will feel stress in the stomach area, and sometimes experience nausea in especially stressful situations.

Early Development and Beliefs

Royal patterning generally develops later at age four to five. As the child grows older, physical intimacy with the parent of the opposite sex becomes confused. This is a time when the appropriateness of taking baths together, lap sitting, or grooming comes into question. The child, sensing the discomfort of the parent, can experience this natural shift in relationship as a rejection of affection and indeed themselves. They are therefore constantly trying to get in the good graces of the parent again, to gain approval and appreciation by behaving and performing perfectly. This need for approval is never completely satisfied and the feeling that they are not good enough leads to an exaggerated drive for accomplishment, such as numerous degrees and other public accolades. This can also be the response to a parent of either sex who expects a child to be independent at an early age – the ability to perform like a little adult is praised. The belief they operate on is "I must be perfect to be loved."

Defenses and Boundaries

Based on their perceived rejection, emotions are uncomfortable and not considered safe. Emotions are also very messy and get in the way of productivity. Cultivating an appearance of perfection in all aspects from dress to performance to social norms, they look to be happy or to have no apparent problems. People are surprised when that "perfect couple" get divorced or the straight A child develops anorexia. The cost of maintaining the appearance of perfection creates a lot of stress and rigidity. They can be anal about rules and regulations to the exclusion of common sense or how others are affected. The Royal energetic and physical boundaries are very *rigid*. Their boundary is like a brick wall, which protects them but also prevents them from truly giving and receiving. All love is conditional. They long to receive and yet their intense boundary prevents it; they have a frozen feeling inside.

Energy Metabolism

Royals have a very controlled and even energy flow, and can easily maintain a strict regimen when it comes to diet and exercise. With all their activity, both work and sports/exercise related, they can burn a lot of calories. It is most helpful for them to have a relaxed mealtime, especially at lunch. The intense amount of energy on the surface of their bodies creates stiffness and tension, which they need to burn off to be comfortable. Massage on a regular basis is very helpful for the Royal. They give little evidence of burnout or exhaustion until they truly shut down; it's an either/or proposition in terms of functioning. They take care of themselves as a practical matter, another thing on their to-do list.

Gifts

The Royals truly are the ones who make the trains run on time and keep all of us on schedule! Their attention to detail and determined focus is so valuable. When their focus becomes disproportionate, they are anxious and fretful; when they are in balance they can design, create, and run anything without sacrificing their emotional lives. When they achieve the balance between Being and Doing, they are exquisitely delicate and even sublime in their expression of love. In receiving love, and being more forgiving of the lack of perfection in themselves and others, they are truly fulfilled.

IDEAL ABODES OF THE ENERGY TYPES...

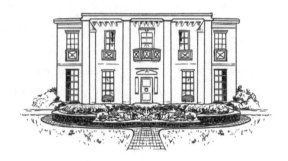

The Royal would create order from a place of power, symmetry, and beautiful proportion. A Colonial Greek style mansion with pillars that can support a great house and a great enterprise, the Royal pays attention and knows how to order the world. Everything and everyone is in its place to perform its perfect function.

BALANCING THE ROYAL

Healthy Guidelines
- Exercise with an aerobic **and** internal calming component like yoga or swimming
- Practice doing – nothing!
- Sense into what you *feel* like doing occasionally

- Meditation to counteract constant Doing and to alleviate stress
- Massage to dissipate physical surface tension
- Intimacy – the combination of love and sex – creates a deeper level of emotional nourishment in relationship

Chakra Focus

- Chakra Energetics: especially the 2nd (abdominal) and the 4th (heart) chakras
- When lying down to sleep, put your hands on your belly and your heart; connecting these two areas will help increase energy in the midline dynamic and calm down the 3rd (solar plexis) chakra

Mirror Mantras

- "I'm good enough"
- "Everything is perfect exactly as it is"

Boundary Work

Softening boundaries is the goal; when tensing up around a situation, bring your breath to your belly with a long exhale.

Stand or sit and visualize your auric field expanding and contracting with your in-breath and out-breath (doesn't matter which direction it goes.) This exercise creates more flexibility in your boundaries (and your diaphragm!)

Visualize expanding your auric field to include your partner when you are intimate.

Antidotes to Defensive Patterns

When dissatisfied and in judgment, notice your personal discomfort and address it – will the world end if something – a person, a project, *yourself* – is not perfect? Notice and soften any hardening that shows up (see expansion/contraction of the auric field in the previous section, Boundary Work).

Do you need to continue to work toward perfection or are you chasing diminishing returns? Look at how much effort you put in the last leg of a project and assess whether it's really necessary. Practice letting go with the breath and your "mirror mantra."

Building on Gifts

The Royal's main issue is ACCEPTANCE. A less obsessive relationship with perfection means cultivating a deep appreciation for the way things are; being comfortable with doing their part and letting the rest be. The Royal is an upstanding individual, an inspiring example of how much we can accomplish with dedication and discipline. When relaxed and in balance, they exhibit strength, compassion, and grace.

PART FOUR

14

Playing Well with Others –
At Home and At Work

R emember that an energy signature is made up of two or
three (or even four) types. It is very helpful to identify
just one and work from there. A person will display
more of the positive attributes of their types if they are self-
aware and growing; likewise they will exhibit the more negative
traits if they are excessive in their energy type patterning.

We are always responding to other people's energy! The
purpose of this book, and especially this chapter, is to help you
make these interactions more *conscious*. We are not trying to
manipulate people into a particular outcome, but to allow a
more productive situation to unfold, naturally. When people
are not in a defensive mode, they can work together better and
more happily. The goal is to bring out the best in everyone!

Understanding the Priest

For a more productive interaction with a Priest:
At work…

- Make eye contact and let them talk first – then it's best to ask a question to focus them on the subject at hand, and go from there.
- Listen carefully for the "nuggets" that may be lost in a long dialogue – be patient with them as they unfold their ideas.
- Be specific about deadlines and expectations; several small deadlines leading up to a big one is best.
- Have regular "idea sessions" in the schedule, with you or another team member; a Priest often processes and formulates their thoughts by talking them out.
- The more convivial the work environment, the better – combined with a solitary space without distractions for concentrated work.
- Complement them on their *ideas* and creative contributions.
- The more aesthetically pleasing the workplace, the better, even if it is just personalizing their own space.
- Have a flexible work schedule – their best working hours may be at night.
- Narrow down options to a few instead of leaving it open-ended; conversely, they can have many responsibilities and projects that they move between, as they like constant stimulation.

- They are idea people who are interested in all the details, but the details shouldn't be their main follow-through function.

At home…

- Touch is the best way to get a Priest's attention! Just a touch on the shoulder can be enough. For more intimate interactions, touch is still the key, starting slowly and building up as they come more into their bodies.
- Let them be the creative designers of the home space but allow for a specific contained area where they can be messy (such as a desk with cabinet doors for a home office).
- Support making an area (and time) for meditation as much a priority as other activities.
- Maintain a stable and reassuring presence.
- Keep a Priest fed and watered – in a restaurant they may have a mostly full plate while everyone else is almost finished (their love of gab…) note this and invite them to eat!
- Don't expect them to do an excessive amount of physical work; Priests tire quickly (the same goes for recreational activity as well).
- As a partner, decide on a plan of action or policy for the household together but do the work/implementation yourself or farm it out. (Priests will do well researching an issue and presenting options.)

- Be aware of and patient with the propensity to be late; they just have a different relationship with time!
- When a Priest is frazzled or overwhelmed, suggest a short time-out such as a walk or a hot bath (maybe they even can have a time-out-of-time menu to refer to).
- Support them by having a household schedule with defined responsibilities for all members.
- The closeness of family members is important and satisfying for a Priest both physically and in communication.

Understanding the Lover

For a more productive interaction with a Lover:
At work…

- They will be the ones to alert you to any emotional undertones going on in a group, whether team members or clients or themselves! Their extreme sensitivity makes them something of a canary in the coalmine for the emotional environment.
- They work best alongside or with others to keep them motivated and engaged.
- They are great interacting with clients but not so great in making demands or handling conflict.
- Encourage and support them but don't let them engage you in long discussions that don't have a point, or take five sentences to say what should be said in one.

- If they are feeling hurt or misunderstood, clarify your intention and ask what they need to move forward.
- Compliment them on the *quality* of their work.
- They are best in roles that are not physically demanding.
- They are aware of and respond to pleasant/unpleasant sensory inputs in the office environment, including cleanliness, smell/scent, and tactile surfaces.
- Be inclusive even when they are not critical to the project, as long as they don't demand too much attention.

At home...

- Lovers need a lot of attention but will return it in spades; like children, they are needy but reciprocal in their affection.
- Do as much as possible together or as a family unit – chores as well as recreational activity.
- If you are doing something that you don't think they would enjoy (that requires a lot of exertion or is unpleasant) always include them while giving them the option to decline.
- Lovers are good at noticing and meeting the needs of others as long as they aren't overwhelmed or ignored.
- Being affectionate, they enjoy pets and are good caregivers.
- They enjoy special treats, personal gifts, and nights out!
- If they are upset or even hysterical, stop and give them your undivided attention – don't rush to a solution or

tell them to get over it; they just need your reassuring presence and/or a hug (and sometimes an apology for their very sensitive hurt feelings).

- Don't minimize their feelings; be respectful but don't add fuel to the fire.
- They are the hypochondriacs of the energy types – if they hear about it, they think they may have it! Don't encourage this kind of thinking; present alternative explanations and shift their attention away from the health focus.

Understanding the Gardener

For a more productive interaction with a Gardener:
At work…

- They are the engines behind a team! Use their consistency of effort to support the overall company/ team.
- They have great physical stamina and strength and can endure harsh conditions.
- They will say yes to everything you ask of them but don't take advantage of this. Promote healthy boundaries, especially if they volunteer without being asked.
- Compliment them on their *efforts* – privately. Check with them about public recognition. They can be shy and not want attention being called to them in public.
- You will need to ask for their verbal input – they can be uncomfortable offering it.

- Over time, you may become aware of some festering resentment about the work, other co-workers, or the boss. Unless you get to the bottom of it the workplace will eventually become poisoned.
- They are dependable and loyal – but once they feel taken advantage of, they will dig in and hold a grudge, silently carry on conversations about what they wished they would have said, and possibly sabotage things.
- They usually won't say "no," they just won't do it! (A warning sign – see above.)
- They will rarely express anger but are the masters of passive aggressive behavior (another warning sign).
- Beware of volunteering and ask yourself if there might be some unspoken reciprocal action that is expected.

At home…

- Gardeners are considerate helpmates and will do more than their share of the heavy lifting.
- Easy going to the extreme, they will accommodate others at the expense of their own needs – they are everyone's best friends! The Gardener's volunteering may frustrate the family when it impacts them negatively.
- In all areas, intimate and otherwise, there is an unspoken expectation that others will know what they need and provide it without any spoken communication. Pay careful attention to subtle hints because that is the most notice you will get!

- Better to clarify their expectations in a situation up front if possible. This will avoid misunderstanding that leads to anger and resentment.

- When your Gardener blows up, know they need help expressing themselves before they reach the boiling point; their anger is often in response to something unimportant, but it is really about a series of events. The anger is often inappropriate to – and not about – the actual incident.

- While physically strong, Gardeners are usually extremely sensitive to touch; they like hugs but go slow and ask for feedback with deeper touch (this is true in massage as well).

- They can be overly emotional and involved in others people's dramas as a way of expressing emotion that is not specific to them.

- They are acutely aware of other people's emotional and physical states and will even *feel this in their own bodies.*

- While their feelings may be obvious to you, they are often unaware of what they are feeling themselves. Encourage them to take time to sense in and report their feelings; if that is difficult for them, focusing on bodily sensations is a good place to start.

- They are generous, sometimes to a fault; don't accept excessive or inappropriate gifts.

- Self-care is ignored until a problem reaches an acute stage. They want to be taken care *of* – they believe if they take care of others, it is automatically reciprocal.

Help them with self-care by drawing attention to their needs and their responsibility for themselves.

Understanding the Warrior

For a more productive interaction with a Warrior:
At work…

- If a subordinate, Warriors still need to be allowed to shine; they are naturally leaders so take advantage of those qualities whenever possible in big and small ways.
- Warriors need to feel in control of a situation; once their control is acknowledged or assured, they are usually more than willing to collaborate.
- Warriors are very sensitive to criticism, so speak thoughtfully about corrections, and definitely not in the presence of others.
- They are willing to take on great responsibility but work best independently or at the head of a group (most leaders in a company have a Warrior component).
- Flattery will get you – somewhere! They are very personable and like to be complimented on any number of things (just make sure you are sincere).
- They are good at assessing complex situations within the big picture; they excel at planning and thinking long-term.
- Warriors are great communicators, for better or worse! They will let you know immediately what is on their mind.

- Co-workers can have strong positive or negative reactions to Warriors; feedback is best channeled to a Warrior via a superior as they can be quite defensive.
- Trust is a main issue, and it often results in a "my way or the highway" approach; make suggestions to "improve," not replace, their plan (even if it ends up changing their plan dramatically).
- They are a big presence and an ideal choice for public speaking and presentations.
- They are excellent salespeople and thrive on competition!

At home...

- Warriors need to be assured of their place as a ruler or co-ruler of the household (this can be problematic with a Warrior child).
- If there are two Warriors in the family, it's best to carve out areas of responsibility but communicate regularly and don't challenge!
- It is hard for them to show any vulnerability or emotion, yet they do feel deeply; comfort silently, and don't overly discuss emotional situations.
- Warriors can seem angry a lot of the time, but remember they express displeasure immediately and then forget about it just as quickly.
- Building trust is of the utmost importance with a Warrior; once that trust is violated it is very difficult to recreate.

- They will carry more than their share of responsibility and are devastated when their efforts fail; they find it difficult to admit failure and will continue trying to make things work if humanly possible.
- Warriors are willing to take risks to achieve their goals; be direct, but not confrontational, if you want information about their means!
- They are naturally looked up to and are attractive and gregarious personalities; understand that they will be in the spotlight most of the time.
- They are good at creating a plan and implementing it for the family/group.
- They need to be appreciated for their efforts.

Understanding the Royal

For a more productive interaction with a Royal:
At work...

- They seek perfection. Give them a playbook and they will execute it flawlessly!
- They work well as a team member but will step into a leadership role if there is a vacuum –whatever it takes to get the job done, right.
- They may have little patience for other people's (lower) standards or even styles of working; ask them to be patient with others as you acknowledge the quality of their work.

- Remember while they may be critical of others, they are the hardest on themselves.
- Always let them know you appreciate their efforts; if you are going to discard some of their previous work, assure them it is not necessarily their fault – it may be because of a change in direction, circumstances, etc.
- They will work 60 hours to get a project 95% good, and keep working more hours to eke out a few more percentage points. Stop them! Congratulate them on being done!
- With respect to diminishing returns; Royals are Energizer bunnies but can eventually burn out or have a sudden major health event. Pace their contributions and workload.
- For a Royal, being on time is being twenty minutes early. Compliment them on their punctuality but don't encourage them in applying that standard to others! (And if you are a Priest-leader, give them the job of setting up for the meeting…)
- They will become extremely frustrated if goals are not clearly defined or keep changing. They want their effort to matter.
- Keep in mind that Royals excel at details unlike any other energy type and they will meet every deadline with excellence.

At home…

- It can be exhausting living with a Royal if you don't have the same desire to be physically active. Do some things together and let them go off on their own or with other friends and family members to engage in their love of extreme sports!
- They are always on the go; this is actually born of a need to release excess tension, so while you may not always participate, encourage their activity or you will have a very stressed Royal on your hands.
- Royals keep emotion at bay because it is such a drag on productivity. They are uncomfortable in emotional territory no matter whose emotions are on display.
- Finding ways to relax with your Royal will help them slow down and get in touch with their inner life; actual touch – like partner massage – is welcome.
- They perform for love, but love them unconditionally!
- They may get upset if family and friends don't follow up on assigned tasks. Help them to be easier with others, and instead of being judgmental, how to creatively motivate others.
- Don't criticize them – encourage them. They are hardest on themselves.
- Just as they like to compartmentalize emotions, the Royal can easily separate love and sex. Be forewarned! In intimate relationships cultivate an appreciation of prolonged sensual contact versus a physical action to

be completed (even if that action is – satisfy partner? Check!).

- Although they may need coaching to slow down and smell the roses, they genuinely aim to please and will be willing to try something different.
- They pride themselves on being responsible and need outward confirmation that they are getting it right.
- They prefer an instruction book or set of rules they can follow to be assured of a specific outcome, and will be quite disappointed if the outcome is not as promised.
- They tend to participate more in organized religion because the beliefs and ideology are clearly defined and demand obedience and execution.

As you work to bring your own energy signature into balance, you will notice changes in the quality of your interactions; with more awareness of other people's signatures, you will enhance those relationships even more. As I embarked on my healing career and started working with my own energy signature, my Warrior-on-Warrior relationship with my father changed and got softer. This was completely unexpected! After forty years I thought our relationship was set in stone, and I certainly was not trying to change him. This was just one of the lovely surprises that came my way as I brought energy awareness into my life.

15

Pitfalls and Progress

O h, if I had only known about energy types and signatures earlier! It was a real wake-up call to the more extreme aspects of my behavior, and how I could improve the way I interacted with others. These insights also helped me work with some of my less desirable habits while at the same time not beating myself up about my shortcomings.

My Warrior tendencies really impacted my kids. The Warrior is the ultimate control freak. When they would do chores, I would "instruct" them on how to do the chore correctly, or better (in other words, *my way*). I thought it was an educational moment; they felt criticized. Ultimately they faced the decision to do the chore and get a "lesson" or to not do the chore and get a scolding. Guess which one they chose? It was also pretty painful to realize that if I always had to be right (and defended any suggestion otherwise) that made my kids – and everyone else – wrong. I had to diligently practice acknowledging they were right, and I was wrong, to counteract that. I still have to keep an eye on these tendencies as they creep back in. Just the other day my Lover daughter (who knows the energy types well) pointed out I was rationalizing (defending) her criticism of my behavior when all she wanted was an acknowledgment and apology.

When I was younger, I joined a non-profit filmmaking group and soon became the Director. Eventually I managed to get everyone to quit (they were volunteers!) because I didn't think they were up to snuff. The only ones I deemed capable were the secretary and treasurer; they came over to my house one day with all the books and resigned because of the way I had treated the others. I was eight months pregnant and on bed rest… and the Warrior in my energy signature had created a nightmare.

As a Warrior woman, I liked dating weak Priest-Lover men (so sweet! so spiritual!) because I could boss them around and be in charge. Eventually I would decide that they were too wimpy and break up. I consciously changed that m.o. and now I can handle the intensity of a Royal or a Warrior who will challenge me.

As a Warrior–Priest it's no surprise that I aspired to and ended up as a Director in my film career. Mid-life I realized I had manifested a perfect Warrior set-up; as a single parent, running my own business both in my energy healing practice and in teaching, I was in charge – of everything. This was no fun. I decided to actively invite partnership into my life (and luckily my Priest loves collaboration!).

Any energy type patterning, when excessive or extreme, is problematic. My unbalanced Priest has gotten me in plenty of trouble too. I remember in college I got an opportunity to make a short film for the newly formed Native American Studies Department. I showed up to a meeting with sketchy handwritten notes – and lots of great ideas! The Department Head dismissed me immediately as disorganized. My Priest patterning was also why I wrote all my college papers the night before. Now I pace myself and prepare ahead of time. Although I still do a final burst, I'm not trying to do an entire project at the last minute. I also try to build in lots of mini-deadlines, preferably with someone else holding me accountable (which is why I finally hired a writing coach to get this book done).

My Priest believes there's always enough money until I realize I'm in trouble (Warrior to the rescue!). As a Priest, not paying enough attention to practical matters like money and time will cause problems and unnecessary stress. I used to always be late, and suffer the complaints of those closest to me. I can't tell you how many times I have been at a dead run through an airport to make my flight (and when I finally actually missed one, for some reason I was shocked).

So while I had lots to work with in my personal life, there were also some learning curves my Warrior–Priest posed for me in my healing practice:

- Priest – time and money boundaries. When I first started, more than once I spent three hours with someone – both of us totally blissed out afterwards – and then I would forget to collect their payment.

- Warrior – the tendency to interrupt, talk too much, and relate my own stories (that wide open 5th (throat) chakra). I literally practiced deep listening, not speaking for several minutes at a time with clients; and during the session review just said what I was guided to (and didn't overwhelm the client with too much information).

There is an upside to your energy signature when you are more in balance (but definitely *not* perfect). I am living a life that is in alignment with the gifts of my Warrior-Priest (Royal) energy signature. I am leading a group, teaching (Warrior) about energy and spirit (Priest) and I have been organized enough to create and run a training program (Royal).

Have you begun to see how you are out of balance, how, where, and why your patterns are excessive, and the cost to you? Don't you want to make it better? Here are some questions to reflect on and see how your energy signature might be affecting your work as a health professional:

- Are you a Royal who gets miffed if your client is late? Are you critical when they don't follow the plan you created for them?
- Are you a Gardener who takes on your clients' energies, even physical aches and pains? Do you do more for your client than is appropriate within the context of the relationship?

- Are you a Warrior who talks more than you listen, who tells your client what to do instead of embarking on a journey of discovery with them?
- Are you a Priest who has a hard time with boundaries and consistency? Senses energy but doesn't know what to do with that information to help your client?
- Are you a Lover who takes comments personally and gets your feelings hurt? Is physical stamina an issue in your practice?

And on the other side of the interaction is your client:

- Are you frustrated with your Gardener client who won't take care of themselves? Do you let your Gardener client take care of *you*, or give you gifts?
- Can you see how your Royal client needs you to be organized and timely to feel comfortable? (Isn't it cute how they will fold up the blankets or even start to change the sheets after getting a massage?)
- Do you get angry with your Priest client for always being late or canceling? Do you let them continue with this behavior or do you hold a boundary?
- Do you let your Warrior client boss you around and tell you what to do? Or even worse, do you argue?
- What do you do with a Lover client who wants you to do everything for them? How do you motivate them?
- If you do bodywork, do you understand the level of touch this client may need to start? (A Gardener will

not tell you if it's too much; a Priest needs deep pressure to even feel their bodies.)

- Which clients will be better able to follow through on a regimen and which ones need reinforcement, encouragement, or reminders?
- What kind and amount of personal attention would make your client feel heard and well served?

I have just scratched the surface of how my energy signature was limiting me, and how I changed those excessive patterns to come into balance and have a healthier, happier, and more successful life. I have developed strategies for working with clients according to their energy signatures and it has really enhanced my relationships and the results of my session work. After learning about energy types, I have become a much better healer, mother, daughter, intimate partner, and friend. My wish is that people would learn about their energy signatures as young adults, and let it inform them as they mature in their relationships and careers.

CONCLUSION

Be an Evolutionary!

B eing able to sense energy fields and forms is an inherent capability within every person. In fact, we all sense energy already, but this information is not conscious – and therefore not readily available to us other than as a "gut" feeling. (The gut is now being referred to as our second brain.) I believe making this information conscious is the next step in human evolution. And this awareness has incredible value in our everyday lives, relationships, and physical health. This knowledge – and the possibilities that it entails – has been known and talked about for centuries, yet is still beyond the grasp of today's average person. You are the one to help bridge this evolutionary gap and take the leap!

Energy signatures are a map of the human physiology which goes beyond personality types to include beliefs, behavior patterns, and the physical body. When you start tuning into the types and signatures, you will see how relevant energy is to our everyday lives. If you are in a healing practice, you will get a direct experience of these energetic patterns and how they form the body. The learning never stops once you step out on this path of increased consciousness and awareness, and life gets way more interesting. I guarantee you it's just the start of a fascinating adventure!

I use my knowledge of energy signatures all the time in the smallest interactions - at the grocery store, or the bank, or just standing in line. It's so easy to guesstimate someone's main signature just from at looking them. Unfortunately, I didn't know about energy signatures when I was a filmmaker; it would have helped when I was being interviewed for a job. On the other side of that equation, I always hired Priests who I got along with famously – and then wondered why they were so flaky! (I finally handed over the hiring of my staff to my Royal producer.) Now this knowledge comes into play when I need support – I want a Royal accountant, a Lover or Gardener babysitter, a Warrior coach. Professions tend to be populated by certain types; doctors tend to be Royal, nurses, Gardeners. Notice how the most successful people are working in fields that employ the gifts of their signature.

Watching movies and assessing the character's energy signatures is one way to get familiar with the energy types. Actors are typecast according to their energy signatures; the manly Warrior, the Lover leading lady (those eyes, those lips!), the Gardener best friend. Another way to practice identifying energy types and signatures is to go to a public place – a coffee shop, library, bar, or restaurant – and just observe. This is really fun to do with a friend (people in my classes bond over this pastime!). Recently I saw a family in a restaurant where you order at the counter and then sit down. The Priest mother immediately went off to order something she forgot; the little four-year old Warrior-in-the-making sat for a moment, then went to get herself a booster seat (without asking for help or even where the seats were located), and wrangled it into her chair by herself. The whole time the Royal dad (sitting across from her) was attending to the 2-year-old Lover's needs. When he tried to leave the table to get water and napkins, the little Lover wailed and he relented (mom still hadn't made it back to the table yet). Now this didn't particularly impact or help me – I didn't interact with the family directly – but it was quite amusing!

Watching yourself as an observer can be helpful in working with your energy signature. Remember to not take yourself too seriously. You are not your patterns; noticing is the first step to change.

As you practice with the types in your own energy signature, you will certainly expand that understanding to those closest to you and eventually everyone you meet. We are not models, but understanding energy signatures is a way to have more compassion for all of us perfectly imperfect humans. This great bazaar of humanity that parades through our lives is infinitely rich and wonderful. The easier you can be with yourself and your shortcomings while making an effort to be better, the more peace and love you will create in the world.

APPENDIX

Chakra Energetics Exercise

An exercise to open and energize your physiology
through your chakra system.
Do the sound and movement of each of the seven chakras,
then return to the first chakra to finish (this helps to
ground and integrate you).
Also included is a description of the specific characteristics
of each chakra: the color/frequency, governing attributes and
issues, and the physical system it is related to.
This is for your information; it's not necessary to know these
things to do the exercise.
By the way, you *will* look silly doing this –
practice being goofy!

FIRST CHAKRA (Base Chakra)
Gorilla Stomp
Movement: Careen around stomping your feet
and hopping occasionally
Sound: Grunting and hooting
(red, bones, physical strength, will to live)

SECOND CHAKRA (Abdominal Chakra)
Hula Hoop
Movement: Rotate pelvis in circles while holding/patting
abdomen; walk with it
Sound: Moaning (in a good way!)
(orange, reproduction, sexuality, emotions, and creativity)

THIRD CHAKRA (Solar Plexus Chakra)
Power Up
Movement: Hands in fists above shoulders, jump several times
while bringing your hands down into your chest
Sound: "I, I, I" (as in me!)
(yellow, muscles, mental activity, ego/identity, and action)

FOURTH CHAKRA (Heart Chakra)
Row Your Boat, Gently…
Movement: Arms extended forward, palms open; close hands
and pull arms back, opening chest
Sound: "Aahhh" (as arms move outward) "Yesss"
(as arms pull back)
(rose/green, circulatory system, personal love, faith)

FIFTH CHAKRA (Throat Chakra)
Open Sesame
Movement: Make a lion's face and do neck stretches
to open and relax
Sound: Slowly tilting head up and down, tone "O"
(blue, digestion, taking in nourishment/information, and
assimilating/expressing it)

SIXTH CHAKRA (Brow Chakra)
Good Vibrations
Sound: Rasping breath - push your tongue against the
roof of mouth with a fast exhale; do several times then stop
(or you will get dizzy)
Movement: After you finish the rasping breath, put your
hands in prayer position; fully rest the weight of your
head on your hands in surrender
(opalescent, nervous system, intuition, relationship with
divine will and divine love)

SEVENTH CHAKRA (Crown Chakra)
Shooting Star
Movement: Reach your hands up to the stars
(on tiptoe if you can) and then bring your hands down to
touch your toes or calves
Sound: "ooohh" (sliding from a high to a low sound)
(gold, endocrine system, connection to spiritual realms)

FURTHER READING

Hands of Light and *Light Emerging* by Barbara Brennan

Eastern Body, Western Mind by Anodea Judith

Your Soul Sings Your Body Dances – Listening to Their Conversation by Dorothy A. Martin-Neville, Ph. D

The Body Reveals – What Your Body Says About You by Ron Kurtz and Hector Prestera, MD

Human Energy Systems Theory by John C. Pierrakos, MD

Character Analysis by Wilhelm Reich

I Feel My Energy Body by Ronda Myer
(Chakra Energetics for children)

ACKNOWLEDGMENTS

So many things contributed to making this book possible! The depth of my understanding of characterology – what I now call energy signatures – would not have been possible without years of practice with my family and students. I especially want to send a shout out to the initial group of students who kept asking for more classes and co-created the School with me – Anne, Frodo, Stephanie, Bob, Rod, Pam, Rich and Genise. My business partner, Stephanie Hull, keeps me and the School up and running; Vicki Wiepking is our media manager, Tamara Leach teaches, Julie Bales is our graphics guru - and all of them are amazing McKay Method healers in their own right. Thanks for putting up with me; I have learned so much from all of you, and continue learning and becoming better every day because of you!

My first teacher was the Inuit healer Della Keats, who was so patient with me, and showed me so much, long before I realized what was going on. We all encounter many wonderful teachers in our lives; for me, many of them come from an energy healing perspective, the Buddhist tradition, or the Indian spiritual heritage. I appreciate them all, but want to recognize in particular Shelby Hammit, Emilie Conrad, Michael Mamas, Byron Katie,

Barbara Brennan, Rosalyn Bruyere, Maharishi Mahesh Yogi, and Sri Aurobindo and the Mother – you all had a major impact on me. I consider myself omnireligious, although after dating Zen Buddhism for decades I finally committed in 2015 (!) This practice has greatly influenced my life and my teaching.

And to those who helped this Priest manifest a book: Angela Lauria, you are my Yoda! After trying for years to write this book, you made real the wisdom of "Do or do not, there is no try!" To my editor Anna Paradox for holding my hand, putting up with my relationship with deadlines, and telling me to stop writing. And to my writing buddies Nurys, Linda, and Maritta – I couldn't have asked for better company on this journey of becoming an author.

To the Morgan James Publishing team: Special thanks to David Hancock, CEO & Founder for believing in me and my message. To my Author Relations Manager, Gayle West, thanks for making the process seamless and easy. Many more thanks to everyone else, but especially Jim Howard, Bethany Marshall, and Nicole Watkins.

Love to my parents, who supported me wholeheartedly; now gone from this earth, they continue to encourage me through our ongoing dialog. Many of my teachers are not in physical form, but still have shown me some great healing techniques over the years – and help me out when I'm in over my head…

And lastly to Ganesh, the Hindu god with an elephant head and human body, who is the Mentor of the School and a tough teacher. He occasionally removes obstacles for me, but mostly gives me the tools to remove my own obstacles!

Ah, and in recognition of the human condition of suffering – we make it so hard for ourselves – that makes us want to do better.

ABOUT THE AUTHOR

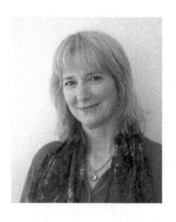

Bear McKay has been in the energy healing field for over fifteen years, practicing, writing, and teaching. She is the Founder and Director of The McKay Method® School of Energy Healing, guiding students for over a decade through a multi-level program to become energy healers. Her simple and direct methods of teaching encompass numerous Eastern, Western and indigenous models of health. Bear's students learn to directly sense energy, employing techniques that affect the entire spectrum of health.

Website: TheMcKayMethod.com

Email: Info@TheMcKayMethod.com

Facebook: Bear McKay/The McKay Method

THANK YOU

You are the Point Person!

Books can be written but will never serve their purpose without you, the reader. I hope I have inspired you to start working with energy signatures, and that it helps you not only understand and work with people better but also to appreciate the mystery of each individual life. I am constantly amazed at what's possible when you begin to notice the energy happening all around us, all the time.

There's more I'd like to share...

Want to support your growing awareness of energy, in very specific ways, in your everyday life?

I'm making available to you my *"Mindfulness and Energy Awareness"* package, which contains a booklet and videos detailing simple techniques for grounding, receiving energetic information, and bringing moments of mindfulness into your

143

day. You'll get to see Chakra Energetics in action and learn how to Hara, an essential beginning point for energy awareness. It's the first thing I teach all of my students and I hope you will learn and use it too!

Download the *"Mindfulness and Energy Awareness"* package from **TheMcKayMethod.com** and get started! It's my small gift to you in appreciation for your efforts to increase your awareness, and to acknowledge the growth in consciousness that **you** are bringing into the world.

Thanks for joining in the adventure – your reality just got a whole lot bigger!

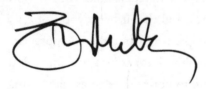

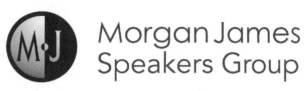

Morgan James
Speakers Group

↗ www.TheMorganJamesSpeakersGroup.com

We connect Morgan James published
authors with live and online events
and audiences who will benefit
from their expertise.

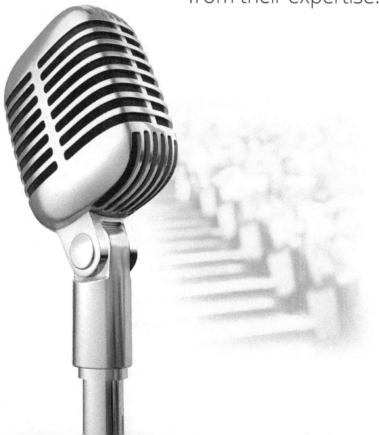

Morgan James makes all of our titles available
through the Library for All Charity Organization.

www.LibraryForAll.org

Printed in the USA
CPSIA information can be obtained
at www.ICGtesting.com
JSHW08234514082 4
68134JS00020B/1896

9 781683 508090